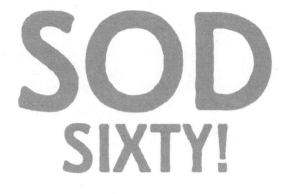

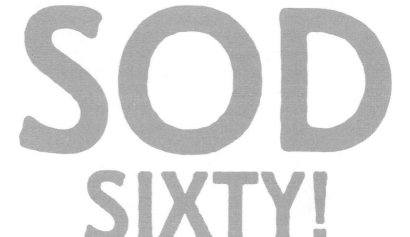

SOD
SIXTY!
THE GUIDE TO LIVING WELL

CLAIRE PARKER
AND MUIR GRAY

BLOOMSBURY

This book is dedicated to Joyce Rosemary Cockram
(11.10.1926 – 17.2.2015) for the inspiration and love she gave to the very end.

Bloomsbury Sport
An imprint of Bloomsbury Publishing Plc

50 Bedford Square
London
WC1B 3DP
UK

1385 Broadway
New York
NY 10028
USA

www.bloomsbury.com

BLOOMSBURY and the Diana logo are trademarks of Bloomsbury Publishing Plc

First published 2016
© Claire Parker, Muir Gray, 2016
Illustrations © David Mostyn, 2016

Claire Parker and Muir Gray have asserted their right under the Copyright, Designs and Patents Act, 1988, to be identified as Authors of this work.

British Library Cataloguing-in-Publication Data
A catalogue record for this book is available from the British Library.

Library of Congress Cataloguing-in-Publication data has been applied for.

ISBN: HB: 978-1-4729-2598-5
ePDF: 978-1-4729-2600-5
ePub: 978-1-4729-2599-2

2 4 6 8 10 9 7 5 3 1

Typeset in Amasis MT by Deanta Global Publishing Services, Chennai, India
Printed and bound in Great Britain by CPI Group (UK) Ltd, Croydon, CR0 4YY

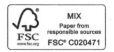

To find out more about our authors and books visit www.bloomsbury.com.
Here you will find extracts, author interviews, details of forthcoming events and the option to sign up for our newsletters.

CONTENTS

PREFACE

Dear Reader

Good health and well-being is not rocket science – they're very simple. Get as active physically and mentally as you possibly can, and then a bit more. It works. Be positive in your approach to the challenges and the opportunities in your life. They all matter.

You really can take charge of your health. It's seldom too late to get fitter and rarely too soon to start doing so. If this is the last line you read then take it away with you – get active and get attitude!

We hope you will find *Sod 60!* fun and helpful. It's all about attitude and action and changing what you think and believe about your health. It's about what you can do to get healthier and stay healthier in your 60s and beyond. And it's about challenging your assumptions – and society's – so that false beliefs about age don't get in your way.

I may be a doctor, but that doesn't mean I've always been as fit as I could be. I knew when I started to think about this book with Muir that I wasn't doing all I could to keep active, not by a long shot. In fact, I knew I couldn't write this book honestly without doing something about my own lifestyle. So last summer I started to get more active, and if I can do it, you can do it.

We have included quite a few 'tried and tested' exercises as examples of the sort of body conditioning and activity levels you should aim for. If you're not yet as active and fit as you might be try these exercises, and you will soon reap the benefits.

This book was inspired by Muir Gray who originally wrote *Sod 70!*, a book about health and well-being for people in their 70s. Muir is a public health doctor – a real mover and shaker of population health care in the NHS in the UK. We take many of his achievements for granted now: his contribution to cervical screening, breast screening, setting up national electronic libraries of health and spearheading easy access to health information for the general public and health professionals alike. Happily his services were rewarded with a knighthood in 2005.

Two particular passions of his have been the health of older people and how we, all of us, make health-related decisions. And so, to celebrate the run-up to his own 70th birthday, he decided to blow apart some of the myths about ageing that stop people keeping active. Hence *Sod 70!*

And this book happened as a direct result of that one along with a twist of serendipity.

It so happens that Muir and I have the same birthday but exactly 10 years apart. We worked together nearly 30 years ago on a project to improve the care of older people with heart disease. At the time we had no idea we shared a birthday, but quite by chance Muir discovered this when celebrating his 70th. So, it was not a complete coincidence but a rather nice twist to the tale when I received an unexpected birthday invitation – not to a party, but to a project to adapt *Sod 70!* for those in their 60s.

But what's so special about being in our 60s that calls for another book? In one sense nothing at all, age is a continuum and it's just by convention that we tend to divide our lives and history into chunks called decades, to handle them more easily. Many of our expectations and life plans tag along with these decade chunks, which do not really reflect natural cycles at all.

It may be that in 20 or 30 years there will be very little detectable difference in health and well-being between our 60s and 70s: and the differences between decades (or even longer intervals) may only start to appear at a much later age.

So why *Sod 60?* Why not use the brilliant *Sod 70!* and make the obvious adaptations in our own mind for the age difference?

Well, we could. And it is more than likely that if someone in the family has a copy of *Sod 70!,* then it might have been read and used by those in their 50s, 60 and 80s, because the fundamental message of 'keep active for better health' is the same, and many of the helpful hints on how to manage health decisions can be applied at any age. But the fact is that '60' is a real transition point, almost a rite of passage in our culture. Not that long ago people whose work was mainly outside the home used to retire at 60 and for women that was the pensionable age. Of course, things have changed, people live longer and many choose or need to work throughout their 60s and into their 70s.

The state pensionable age has been 65 for some years and is creeping higher as life expectancy increases. Women of the class of 1954, will currently collect their state pension at about 67 and can, on present trends, expect to live at least another 20 years or more. For those who have chosen to retire from their first main occupation at 60, as I have done, it's often seen as a time to change career or the direction of it rather than to stop working altogether.

So because 60 is often seen as a significant turning point in life with many years ahead, it is a real opportunity to seize the moment and take stock of our health and well-being.

We hope this book will help you seize the moment and take charge of your own well-being, so that with a bit of luck in avoiding those diseases that can take any of us by surprise, you will be even fitter at 70 than you are at 60. And should 'Stuff Happen' and diseases or unwelcome life events come your way, the aim of this book is that you will be more resilient to cope with them and fitter to manage them.

So here is *Sod 60!*, from us to you.

Claire Parker and Sir Muir Gray

GETTING OLDER DOESN'T MATTER: GETTING ACTIVE AND GETTING ATTITUDE DOES

The good news as you enter your 60s is that whatever your life history so far – your genes, family background, upbringing and unique life experiences, whether or not you have medical conditions that need special care, it is seldom too late to get more active or to soon too start.

Sod 60! is about 'being' as well as 'doing' and 'attitude' as well as 'action'. It's about getting more active. What has past is past, and we can learn from it. The future hasn't happened. We can think about it, plan it and imagine it, but we can really only focus our attention where we are right now.

This book is about how you can take charge of your health and make the most of your 60s and beyond. It explores false assumptions about ageing which can creep up before you realise. You can overturn these before they inhibit your fitness and your independence.

But this book is *not* 'a rosy gloss' on the realities of life. It's not a numbing or a dumbing of problems that might exist and it doesn't pretend that self-help can achieve everything. Difficulties and diseases do occur. *Sod 60!* is based on the understanding that Stuff Happens in life. But neither is this book fatalistic. It's about well-being in our ordinary lives, with all their ups and downs.

Ageing and disease are different processes, even though they sometimes co-exist. Both fare better if we can keep as active as we possibly can. The evidence is overwhelming: activity is central to fitness and fitness is fundamental to well-being – even if we have a medical condition.

Physical strength and mental resilience are more closely connected than you might think. They help each other, and both together help you to struggle through a nasty bout of flu as well as cope with the ups and downs of life. So fitness and resilience are a strong combination, and underpin your health and your well-being.

Getting fitter and staying fitter improves the outcome of many diseases that can occur in later life. And the evidence is strong – research shows that this applies to cancer, heart disease, diabetes, arthritis, depression and, very possibly, dementia.

Good health and well-being should be open to everyone. They are your true wealth and can be shared.

How this book is arranged

Each chapter focuses on a different aspect of your well-being. Some pearls of practical wisdom are scattered through the chapters – a 'string' of interludes that act as little boosts and reminders to add to your mental and physical toolkit – to use now or to file away for future use.

Here is Pearl No. 1. Provided you can stop what you're doing for a few moments, here is a simple series of stretching and balancing exercises that can start getting you fitter and help you feel good right away. First check that the surroundings are safe (if you've had a recent operation, fracture or heart attack, it's best to check with your GP that it's safe to do them). If you feel any pain or twinges, stop the stretch. (There are more exercises to try in Chapter 2.)

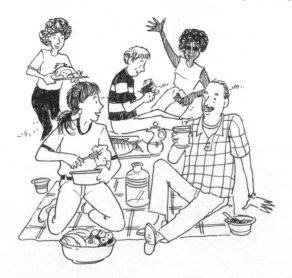

PEARL NO 1. STRETCHING 60!

Stand straight and tall with your feet firmly on the ground. Breathe naturally throughout. It's a simple routine, and you can turn to it anytime. Here goes:

✓ Stretch up each arm alternately, as high as you can, pointing your fingers and stretching those muscles each side of your torso as you do. Hold for a few seconds at the top of the stretch. Repeat five times each side. The movement should be fairly slow and gentle – no thrusting.

✓ Keeping your head straight and level, gently rotate your neck, a semi-circle to the left, back to centre, then to the right, and back to centre. Each time, look as far back over your shoulder as you comfortably can. Hold for a few seconds. Repeat five times each side.

✓ Pull your shoulders back as far as you can, with your arms hanging loosely by your side, so you feel the muscles between your shoulder blades working. Hold for five seconds, then relax completely. Repeat ten times.

✓ With your hands on your hips, rotate your waist to bring your upper torso round to the left as far as you can go. Give a little extra push to the rotation at the end of the stretch. Then do it to the right. Repeat five times each side.

✓ With legs apart and hands clasped behind your head: bend sideways, a couplet to the left, back to centre, then a couplet to the right, and back to centre. Five times each side.

✓ Stand near a wall or table for support if you need it. Stand on your right leg, and bend up your left leg at the hip with your left knee bent. Hug it for a few seconds. Then repeat on the other side. Stand squarely on the floor between each move. Repeat five times each side. If you don't feel steady on your feet, don't do this one.

This shouldn't hurt, but you should feel that you've gently stretched some muscles that you might not have used for a long time.

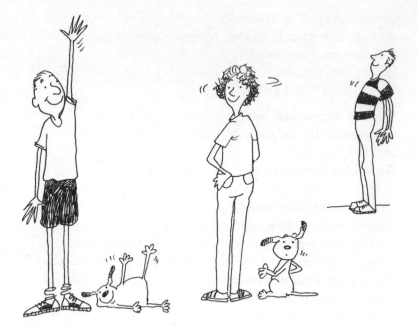

Here are some statistics reported by Age UK and the Academy of Medical Royal Colleges in 2015:

- Nearly 1 in 5 of everyone currently living in the UK is likely to live to 100 years.
- At 65, the UK life expectancy is about 86.1 years for women and 83.6 for men.
- There are over 14 million people aged 60 or over, more than the under 18s.
- Less than one third of UK adults over 65 do the minimum activity for good health.
- Two thirds of women and more than three quarters of men aged 65+ are overweight.
- 3.8 million people 65+ (more than a third of over 65s) live alone, 70 per cent of them are women.

But it's not just how long you live that counts, but how good those years are. Hitting 60 now you can expect over 25 more years if you're a woman and nearly 25 if you're a man. But you might have 40 and make it to 100. So it's a good plan to make the years ahead the best you can, whatever your starting point.

Your 'health span' is as important as your lifespan and your lifestyle makes a huge difference to it, whether or not you have a medical condition. You may have your own list of what you've found important for your well-being and health, but here is *Sod 60*'s Spectacular Seven (discussed in more detail in Chapters 2, 3, 4 and 5):

1. **Be true to yourself**: and find your purpose in life.
2. **Keep as active as you can, physically and mentally**, and keep on keeping active.
3. **Keep connected and be generous with others**: you matter to people and they matter to you.
4. **Find your healthy weight**: up with your Mediterranean diet – vegetables, fruit, fibre, wholegrains, oily fish and vitamin D, and down with sugary drinks, biscuits, cakes, pastries, pies and processed meats.
5. **Keep your alcohol within safe limits**, and **quit smoking**.
6. **Check your blood pressure** and keep it under control.
7. **Bust stress** and practise mindfulness.

We're in our 60s: but who are 'We'?

Claire's friend Marion went on a walking holiday to celebrate her 61st birthday earlier this year. When she asked her where to send her birthday card she laughed and said she thought she might stop remembering her birthdays from now on – unless she could slice a year off her age instead of adding one on. And there you have it. Why shouldn't we feel fitter at the end of the year than when we started it? What does age matter?

Your date of birth is one of the first labels society attaches to your identity. It follows you through life and most important documents you sign require it. But chronological age is simply the number of years since the day of your birth. It doesn't determine who you are. You, with your life history and life choices, define the person you are and want to be.

The era of your birth, together with your genetic inheritance, family background and environment are factors influencing your early life, growth and development. They play a role in your health potential and life expectancy. These major factors do not define the person you are, however – you can do this.

Which brings us to a fascinating question: who are we, and what is special about those of us in our 60s in the early 21st century?

Firstly, many of us experience living in what might be described as a 'squeezed middle'. Many of us have at least one surviving parent. Some of us are carers for elderly parents living into their late 80s or 90s. At the same time, we may have continuing responsibilities to older children if we started childrearing later in our reproductive life, or help with the care of grandchildren so their parents can continue working. These responsibilities exist alongside the transitions of our work, career, changing or lost relationships, and the individual circumstances of our physical, mental and social well-being. Every day can feel like a complicated balancing act with a sense of 'not much time' left over. We can feel 'squeezed' in the middle of all this.

Secondly, we are the class of post-war children. There were major changes in our parents' world. If you're currently in your 60s you'll be in the first wave of post-war baby boomers. If you're in your 50s, you'll be in the second wave. In Britain, at the start of the baby boom, our parents were still living with wartime rationing, and a 'just enough' expectation of food supply. Some of us had parents who had only just arrived in the UK. Cars and TVs were rare. Most people walked or cycled and took the bus or the train for longer journeys. By the mid- to late-1950s, when the first wave of baby-boomers were still at primary school, rationing had gone and cars, fast food and TVs were flooding in big time. It was a perfect storm for unfitness, 50 to 60 years later.

More driving – less walking; more TV – less talking; more sweetened drinks, biscuits, chocolates, crisps and deep-fried fast foods, less vegetables and home-cooked stews and fish. Unfortunately, most households placed a tub of salt on the kitchen table – bad news for our blood pressure 30, 40 and 50 years later. Smoking was widespread throughout the war years and children suffered passive smoking, especially on long journeys in small cars. Bad luck us.

Lifestyle and health

Over the decades since the 1940s and 50s there has been a huge amount of research into the causes of common diseases, such as heart disease, cancers and 'late onset' (now called type 2) diabetes. As the studies poured in, the evidence piled up and quite a few pennies began to drop. The more inactive we are, the less healthy we are. A sedentary lifestyle at home and at work was a recipe for ill health.

Sir Richard Doll was a dedicated medical researcher, working from the 1950s right up to his death in 2004. In the late 1950s he was the first to prove that smoking was the major cause of lung cancer. His life and research inspired thousands of others, not least doctors, who gave up smoking in droves following the publication of his research.

In the 1970s a connection was noticed between high salt intake and high blood pressure and in 1994 departments of health in the UK and internationally advised people to stop adding salt to their food to help them prevent it. Since the 1990s, obesity and lack of exercise have been found to be major factors in the epidemic of type 2 diabetes and, hand in hand with smoking, major contributors to heart disease and atherosclerosis (clogging up of the arteries, see Chapter 5, page 109).

And let's not forget stress, the pressures of working, raising a family, coping with not much money and how to make it go round. It drives up smoking, excess alcohol, comfort eating and addictions. Stress is a major contributor to ill health: from anxiety and depression to stomach ulcers and heart attacks.

Things have been slowly changing. Over the last 15–20 years people have been waking up – and walking more. Fitness classes have sprung up offering activities from gentle stretching to Pilates, Tai Chi, yoga and Zumba for people in their 50s and beyond – and they're catching on.

The message is getting through. A recent study in Ireland found that nearly 70 per cent of the over 65s in that population reported doing the recommended amount of moderate exercise (see Chapter 2). And the less time a person spent sitting, the more likely they were to clock up their activity throughout the week. So the take home message is, don't chain yourself to your chair.

But many of us haven't grasped the nettle and are still locked into bad habits for health. How is this, given that we are absolutely bombarded with information? The short answer is that information, important though it is, isn't enough to change our behaviour.

Putting evidence into action: It's attitude we need

How do we change ourselves? How do we change our habits? How do we turn information into action? Changes to the law can help with some aspects of health (such as the ban on smoking in public places), and campaigning for change is vital – especially to reduce the amount of hidden sugar in drinks and processed foods. But why wait for this to happen? Not everyone wants to go to exercise classes or can afford to, however effective they are. The key to changing our actions is our attitude: Attitude with a big 'A'!

A surprising source of 'Attitude'

We can often look to people we know – in our family or among our friends and acquaintances – whose examples can really inspire and touch us. Take Father Christmas, for example.

FATHER CHRISTMAS

Claire's dad was 90 on Christmas day. His second name? 'Noel'. He had three heart attacks in 30 years and his coronary arteries were too blocked up to allow stents in (tiny tubes to keep the arteries open). So he manages angina with tablets and his arthritis by 'keeping on the go'. He quit pipe smoking years ago. He amplifies poor vision with magnifiers and his 'glasses plus', a pair of toilet rolls taped on to the lenses, to reduce glare from overhead lights.

Despite all this, he was Carer No. 1 for Claire's mum, a talented, active, outgoing lady until the last few years of her life. He organised a complicated but efficient care plan.

On top of all this he played the organ (with a full range of stops) in the front room – and still does. He still has a wonderful network of friends whose support is invaluable.

Claire asked him how he kept going and what his advice might be for someone rather younger – someone turned 60 like her! His answer was immediate and surprising.

He tapped his head. "You've got to have the right **attitude** – be positive and keep your mind **active**". He indicated the world around him with a typically Dickensian flourish: "You've got to get what's in your head out here, into the world – you've got to make your ideas work and make them active". What more could she ask!

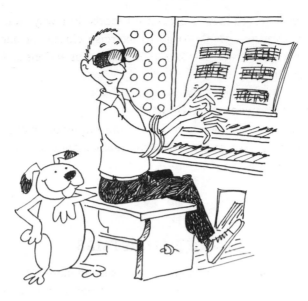

Becoming yourself: Liberation from 'the Norm'

What is normal? Living well is often about overcoming assumptions, as Francesca Martinez, a stand-up comedienne (with Attitude!) has shown. She overcame her inhibitions about her cerebral palsy, her 'wobblies' as she called it, and made them part of her career for everyone to see.

She realised that we all have imperfections, so there's not much point fixating on them. She decided to embrace her 'wobblies'. Awesome.

Overcoming obstacles, developing resilience and a 'can do' attitude, are helpful for young people and people of any age. It helps in our 50s and 60s and on into our 70s and 80s, even if we have medical problems. And the goal of this book is to help you!

What is health and where does fitness fit?

Health

One of the first things the World Health Organization (WHO) did when it was formed, just after the Second World War, was to come up with a definition of the word: **Health is a state of complete physical, mental and social well-being and not merely the absence of disease or infirmity.**

What's interesting is that this doesn't refer to age at all and applies right across social and cultural divides. It gets straight to the heart of the matter.

It makes clear that health is not just the absence of something negative (disease), but the presence of something positive – a state of total well-being in itself.

Fitness enhances health and well-being

Fitness is about our emotional and social health as well as our physical. And physical fitness has many facets too, as we shall see in Chapter 2. It plays a huge role in our well-being.

We do age. Diseases do happen and we all need a bit of luck to avoid those that aren't preventable.

You may say, very reasonably, that older people who are active, robust and full of life are 'able to be fit' because they are healthy, rather than the other way round. That is a good point and sometimes true. There are plenty of long-term studies which apply to people in their 50s, 60s and 70s, which show the link of cause and effect; increasing one's level of fitness leads to an increase in health and well-being.

Fitness helps prevent many diseases and their complications

Long-term studies also show that when fitness improves, the risk of preventable diseases is reduced. This is called **primary prevention**.

Amazingly, getting active and keeping active, stopping smoking, eating healthily and losing weight if you need to can all contribute to a reduction in the risk of *complications* of these conditions as well. This is called **secondary prevention** and is a wonderful way of reducing the 'burden' of disease you might already have.

Attitude active into action

Do **ASK** if you're not sure how to take action to get fit with the condition(s) you may have. GPs often find their patients are their best teachers. They often show how simple measures, such as exercise and keeping fit, can improve well-being and quality of life – even in the face of significant illnesses and ongoing medical problems.

A POSITIVE PATIENT

Claire recently recognised a former patient by her colourful walking stick. She'd recently developed a chest condition called COPD (chronic obstructive pulmonary disease) and had been prescribed regular exercise classes. When she turned around she was radiant – far from a picture of ill health. 'It's been the best thing that's ever happened to me,' she said. 'I feel so much better. I'm going to pulmonary rehab classes and I do weight training and treadmill exercises *twice a week*. **I have to do the exercises every day** otherwise their effects wear off but I feel marvellous. *It's the best thing that's ever happened!'*

Step up your attitude: what you believe matters

Your goals and what life means to you are what get you up in the morning. Your beliefs matter and your choices are the ones that count. The values you put on different lifestyles, and the health outcomes that might follow them, are not necessarily the same as mine or your friends. Rudolf Nureyev famously said: 'You live as long as you dance'. But no 'one size' fits all.

Research into how we perform has shown that if you believe you can do something, and are capable of it, you are more likely to succeed than when you don't believe it. And if we look at examples of people who radiate health *and* take account of the evidence accumulating from long-term studies of fitness and well-being we find that, whatever our age, as our fitness improves so does our health – now and also in the future. And this is *especially* true as we get older.

Where attitude acts

How often did people tell you you needed to 'slow down' as you headed towards your 60s? And if so, how often did you feel confident enough to say: 'slow *what?*' or better still, '*balls!*' in reply?

Great if you did! But if you didn't, you would not be in the minority.

Sometime in our adult life we seem to slide from thinking we can do something about how fit we are into a much more passive acceptance of our body condition. Perhaps it starts to happen as far back as our early 30s. We start to behave as if our body will take care of itself and eventually, by the time we're in our 50s and 60s, we blame our age when it doesn't.

False assumptions

If you have tended to slow down and reduce your physical activity because you assume that's what you should do as you get older, then your fitness and consequently your health will suffer. You will need to counter your assumptions radically and make sure your attitude is on your side.

TWO FALSE ASSUMPTIONS

1. I'll carry on being able to do all the ordinary things I've always done (stepping down and getting up again, keeping upright, looking over your shoulder, pulling up your tights, putting on a heavy coat, tying your laces or running for the bus).

2. I won't be able to do the more demanding things I used to do because of my age.

The reality is:

1. If you take **no action** you may **not be able** to do things in the future that you take for granted now.

2. If you **take action** you **will be able** to do many of the things you assume your age will prevent.

Getting older

Most of us don't feel 'old' as we enter our 60s because the lives we live just don't fit with the notion. But our bodies are changing. Does ageing matter? How does it relate to diseases that we link with it? Where does fitness fit in?

As we answer these questions we will discover what the real problem with getting older might be, and it's not 'ageing' itself.

Ageing is universal

Our everyday expressions give us many clues. How about these for starters: 'He's 65 but has the body of a 40-year-old', 'She's only 60 but she looks 10 years older', 'Gosh you look 10 years younger now you've changed your job', and so on.

Expressions like these show three things. Firstly, there are changes we recognise in most people with the passage of time, and we call them 'ageing'. These are so universal they can be thought of as 'natural'. We recognise them in other animals too. What causes ageing and what might be done about it are quite different questions.

Secondly, chronological age alone does not determine our 'physiological' age – in other words the age our bodies behave and look like. And thirdly, the onset of 'ageing' varies between people.

The last two observations are fascinating and important. They suggest that there are things that can influence the rate and nature of the ageing process and that we ourselves might be able to influence the rate of it even if we cannot reverse it.

Natural ageing processes

By the time we are in our 60s most of us have noticed some changes. Our hair goes grey. We notice more lines and creases in our skin and a slight loss in its elasticity and tautness. Our joints get stiffer quicker with inactivity and our balance is not so hot. Our reaction times are slightly slower, and we have to 'fish around' longer to retrieve things from our memory.

These changes are so common that we consider them 'ageing' rather than disease processes. You can manage, counteract or compensate for most of these by taking simple measures to care for your body and keep it well conditioned (see Chapter 5).

Two examples of age-related changes that affect both men and women are Age Related Hearing Loss (ARHL), and difficulty adjusting visual focus (presbyopia). Both of these conditions can be compensated for, with a hearing aid or varifocal spectacles as appropriate.

These are useful examples because they demonstrate that sometimes the best way to deal with a problem is to find a practical solution to it quickly, so that quality of life is not impaired. This attitude works well for *many* conditions, whether or not they are age-related, and reflects a positive approach, which helps foster and maintain well-being. Unfortunately, we don't always use the help available (see Hearing, Chapter 5 page 97)

The gender divide

There is an obvious, naturally occurring difference between the sexes: women have a menopause, the average age of which is about 52. In contrast to men, whose hormone levels fall gradually, women's hormone levels fall relatively dramatically over a matter of months. The drop in oestrogen levels contributes to a greater loss of bone and muscle strength, and connective tissue changes, than would otherwise occur more gradually with age (see Chapter 4 page 74, Chapter 5 page 125, and Chapter 6 page 146).

The onset and impact of the menopause varies. However, it is often seen as a 'rite of passage' into a woman's middle life.

For many women, though not all, getting to the other side of the menopause is a liberation, and many of the hormone-related changes can be counteracted by a more active lifestyle change, changes of attitude and sometimes medication. Hormone Replacement Therapy (HRT) is used much less frequently by those of us in our 60s than a decade or so ago, because of concerns about increased risk of breast cancer and circulatory problems. But recent guidelines from the National Institute of Health and Care Excellence (NICE, www.nice.org.uk) on managing the menopause help women make more informed decisions about the balance of benefit and risk acceptable to them.

Ageing in context

It's worth putting ageing itself into the context of our life. Usually we think of it as a phase that starts after our physical maturity has peaked (see Figure 2 on page 16) and this approach is useful in helping us understand what we can do to improve and maintain our health as we enter our 60s, or even before. But the reality is that, in some ways, we are ageing from the moment we are born.

What we often fear about ageing is the seemingly inevitable link with disease – even though we know from examples and studies that many people continue to be healthy as they get older, and some die in very old age without having any identifiable disease.

Our main fear is dementia (though it is relatively rare in our 60s). We are *not* usually reassured when we notice minor memory changes, however common we are told they are, because we fear their progression. But knowing a little about the background to these common changes can help us understand that age-related memory loss and dementia are not the same – even though we may not know what exactly is going on in either (see Chapter 5).

But the multi-million dollar question still remains, what causes the ageing process?

What causes ageing?

The honest answer is: we really don't know. It is likely to be complex and to reflect fundamental biological processes going on inside our body tissues, especially in those cells that can divide to replace others that have worn out.

Ageing is also influenced by many of the factors that make us unique: our genetics, our environment. And it is increasingly clear that how active we are and the quality of our diet are important factors in age-related change and, perhaps, the ageing process itself.

So we know quite a bit about the factors *associated* with ageing, as well as some of the actions we can take to offset its effects – even if we don't know precisely how they work. But we needn't let what we **don't** know obscure what we **do** know.

And the evidence is overwhelming. If we increase our activity (see Chapter 2), keep a healthy weight and adopt a Mediterranean diet rich in olive oil, coloured vegetables, fruit and oily fish, it helps heart, circulation and 'metabolic health' (see Chapter 4 page 75), and can improve brain function. Research shows that regular brisk walking in our 50s, 60s and 70s is associated with an increased volume of grey matter as well as an improvement in our thinking skills. Some experts have even suggested that walking might stimulate the brain to recruit and grow new nerve cells – something that traditionally was never thought possible.

The conundrum of age and disease

Most people, including doctors, view ageing and disease as different processes, but they often co-exist and there are some processes where the boundaries are more blurred, such as inflammatory and autoimmune conditions.

In our society sudden deaths are much less common than the diseases that gather with age. Many of us live with 'continuing conditions': coronary heart disease, type 2 diabetes, respiratory diseases, arthritis and even cancers.

On the surface of it, chronological ageing *is* associated with these things. Illnesses and disabilities do accumulate with increasing years of life and it is a fact that, in Western society, 'ageing' (rather than infectious disease, malnutrition and trauma) is the most common risk factor *associated* with death. So how can we unlock this particular puzzle?

Although ageing is associated with disease it is not usually its cause, and is rarely the actual cause of death until extreme old age is reached. The other obvious point is that as the proportion of older people in society increases, age is bound to feature as an increasingly common *association* with death. With time, the risk factors that are the true causes of disease have had longer to act. The most important examples are smoking-related diseases, obesity related illnesses such as type 2 diabetes, and the effects of high blood pressure that is not well managed.

Our growth and decline: Where did all the fitness go?

Ability, fitness and slowing age-related decline

We can use a simple diagram to understand a bit more about the ageing process, and can also use it to see how fitness 'fits in':

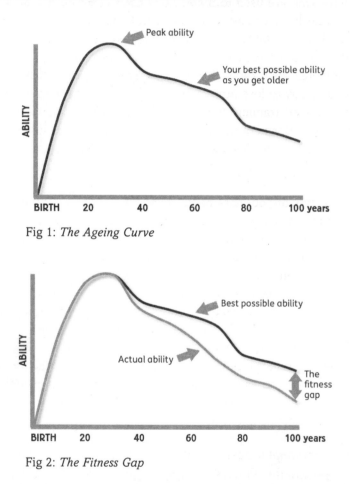

Fig 1: *The Ageing Curve*

Fig 2: *The Fitness Gap*

Figure 1 shows how our 'best possible' ability changes from birth to death. It shows the effect of age alone, and illustrates the best possible pattern of change for most of the physical and mental abilities we have. There are two phases. First, there is a phase of growth in ability from birth to maturity, then a more gradual, prolonged phase of decline from maturity to death, due to age-related loss of ability year by year. The turning point, where our ability peaks, is usually in our early 30s or even before.

The exact timing and size of the peak varies between people even when they are performing at their best possible level, because of individual differences reflecting nature and nurture, experiences and environment during childhood and early adult life.

Athletes who are used to maintaining their best possible ability know that once they have 'peaked', training cannot completely overcome a slight age-related loss of ability, year on year. This is why there is a characteristic 'peak age' for record-breaking in most sports and activities.

But athletes also know that even past their peak, once they stop training and start to lose fitness, they lose their ability more quickly than if they continued training. Inactivity leads to much more rapid decline. Various top performers, including the pianist Paderewski, have been credited with the following quote: 'If I miss one day's practice I know it. If I miss two days, my teacher knows it. And if I miss three days, the public know it.'

Most of us in our 60s have been nowhere near our best ability since our early adult life. With age, we lose ability more quickly the less active we are and the less practice we have.

But we don't have to be athletes or top performers to be 'able'. Even in the absence of disease (but especially in its presence) declining fitness contributes to more rapid decline in ability than age alone can account for. In fact, our 'ability' could just as well be referred to as our 'fitness'.

But as we can see in Figure 2, the rate of decline can vary within a person. You can regain fitness as well as lose it and if you keep on regaining fitness over time you can reduce your rate of decline, and keep yourself 'able' for longer. And you can do this at almost any age, all the way from 30 to 90: and most definitely in your 60s.

Your own personal fitness gap and how to close it

This brings us to the 'Fitness Gap', shown in Figure 2. It is the difference between your actual ability and the ability you could have. If you are not as fit as you could be, but take action to get fitter, you can begin to close this gap and, if you keep getting fitter, you can reduce the rate of your decline.

It is surprising how quickly the fitness gap can close relative to your lifespan. It can happen over weeks and months, and the effect of this is to increase your 'health span'. It does take a little while. But many people say they feel better almost immediately. Measurable fitness – our stamina, endurance, skill and suppleness – can improve over a matter of weeks and months, as we shall see in Chapter 2.

Disease impacts on ability: but finding fitness rescues much of it

It is absolutely true that diseases and continuing medical conditions can affect your ability. But long-term studies exploring cause and effect have shown that improving fitness usually improves the progress of medical conditions, with very few exceptions.

In the case of heart disease, and especially after a heart attack, it is important to get personalised advice on what kind of activity and how much of it is safe for you to do, and at what rate you can safely build up your level. The benefits of increasing exercise need to be weighed against the slightly increased risks during exercise itself. Gradually increasing your exercise tolerance is part of rehabilitation and treatment, and always needs to be discussed.

You have to accept that you cannot relive years that have passed. But the good news is that whatever your starting point, it need not govern your future. Almost always you can get more active, reduce your fitness gap and slow your decline.

Disability, by definition, impacts on ability

Disability, like disease, has many different causes, not all of them preventable by lifestyle. It may be lifelong, the result of birth injury, trauma, accident, or disease later in adulthood. If you have a disability, hidden or visible, it is likely to have had a profound effect on your freedom, health and well-being, needing effort and determination to overcome the limitations imposed.

You need help to find exercise that's suitable and realistic to maintain and increase your fitness. And it's worth remembering that fitness is friendly. Getting fitter works well with all the other things you may need to do to ensure your disability doesn't get the upper hand.

In fact, it is when you have disability or disease that you really need every bit of fitness you can find to close your fitness gap as much as possible. If your condition is more advanced, you may need rehabilitation therapy with carefully graded exercise.

Does fitness have a limit?

You might see a steady fitness level throughout your life. There is still a limit to how much we can improve our physical fitness, even if we give it our best shot and keep going, because of that tiny loss in maximum potential capacity year on year. But most of us never get near our fitness potential as we get older.

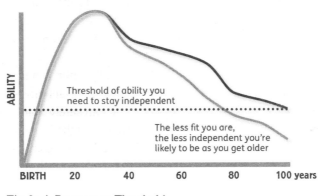

Fig 3: *A Dangerous Threshold*

A dangerous threshold

Figure 3 shows what can happen if the fitness gap doesn't close.

The bottom line shows us that this person was able and active in her early 30s, but became significantly unfit over time. Her lifestyle was almost completely sedentary and car-bound, and she became overweight. Her joints were stiff and painful to walk on, she found it difficult to bend down and put on her shoes and walking the short distance to the bus was a considerable effort. In other words she was losing her independence.

But the top line shows that if she had got more active, lost weight and gradually closed her fitness gap year-by-year during her 60s, she would have climbed towards the fitness potential that she could have expected at the age of 70 with the prospect of remaining active and independent until well into her early 80s.

We can still encourage her, of course, because we know that as she heads into her 70s, she can still get active, lose weight and improve her fitness as much as she can. But it would have been better if she had arrived at 70 even fitter than she was at 60.

Are you finding fitness, or losing it rapidly, as the years tick by? If your fitness gap widens year on year you are at risk of a more rapid loss of independence.

Two pathways

Growing older can go hand in hand with greater fitness, more well-being, less disease and healthier ageing, as summed up in this little diagram:

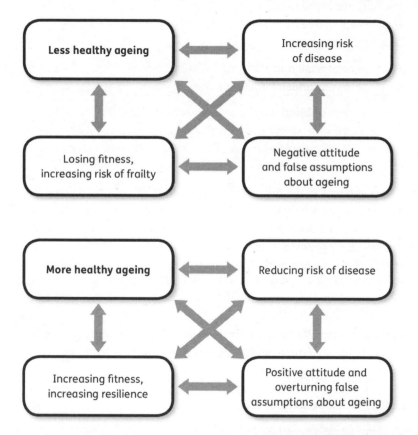

Fig 4: *Growing Older: Less Healthy or More Healthy? How Fitness and Attitude Fit In*

Make the decision to stay active in your 60s and beyond, and do it now.

This book is about what you can do to reduce your fitness gap and improve your health and well-being through your 60s and into your 70s. If you get fitter and stay fitter you are much more likely to feel better and maintain your independence for years to come. If you're already doing enough physical and mental activity – please keep going. If not, you may be in the majority but it's a dangerous comfort zone.

SO, SOD 60! You *can* step up your attitude *and* keep active!

Here's Pearl No. 2.

PEARL NO 2: THE MINDFUL MIRROR

The purpose of the mirror is to accept your body as it is – so you can engage with it, free from angst, while you get more active and get your body fit for purpose.

You also need a tall mirror in a warm, private room where you can stand naked or in your underclothes.

If you can think objectively about your weight you may not need this mirror. But if your weight makes you unhappy this can be difficult. And if you think you have a serious problem at either end of the weight scale, please discuss this with your doctor.

Before you look in the mirror remember that, whatever your shape or size, your body is your very own. Accept yourself as you are now. Being more or less fat doesn't make you more or less good. You don't need punishment or reward. If you need to change your weight to improve your health – it's just a job. Get on with it non-judgementally. It's your decision, not a punishment. Don't beat yourself up.

When you're ready, have a look at yourself in the mindful mirror.

Continue doing this for two or three minutes. Be still within yourself. Then ask yourself three questions, breathing slowly all the time:

1. **'Am I overweight?'**

2. **'Can I pick up folds of fat easily?'**

3. **'Am I apple-shaped** (with fat building up mostly around my tummy) **or pear-shaped** (with fat more on my hips and thighs)?

Register your answer, and breathe slowly.

Let your answers rest in your mind and accept them. Consider the following: if your first two answers were yes, you are likely to be overweight. If your third answer was 'apple-shaped' (due to fat tissue in and around your tummy) then you are significantly overweight and will benefit from losing it. You risk overloading your joints, heart and metabolic system (see Chapter 4).

But don't be anxious – be relieved that you're going to tackle the problem slowly but surely. Gradual is great and sustainable: go with it. As time goes on you may want to use your scales as well for accuracy. But make friends with yourself and your mirror first: it's a good partnership to start with.

2

KEEPING ACTIVE IS FITNESS FRIENDLY

Exercise and fitness

Q: What do they look like?
A: A bit sweaty, a bit puffy and Absolutely Fabulous!

You are in your 60s and can set fitness free. You don't need money, or lycra or fancy trainers. You just need to know that **you can do it**, whoever you are, wherever you are and whatever has happened in your life so far.

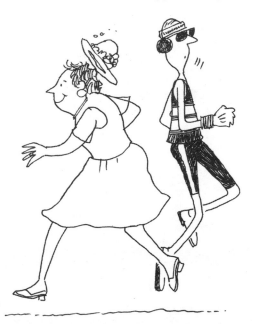

Exercise

In 2015, the Academy of Medical Royal Colleges were so bowled over by the weight of evidence for the benefit of just 30 minutes of sweaty, puffy exercise five times a week, that they published a report about it. They called it 'Exercise – the Miracle Cure', and here are some of its findings:

Regular exercise at the recommended level …

- reduces the risk of breast cancer by as much as 25 per cent
- reduces the risk of bowel cancer by as much as 45 per cent
- reduces the risk of ever developing dementia by as much as 30 per cent
- reduces the risk of ever having a stroke by 30 per cent
- reduces the risk of developing heart disease by OVER 40 per cent.

Considering how common these conditions are in people aged 65 and above (in 2015, there were over 2 million people with coronary artery disease, over 700,000 with dementia and over 100,000 with stroke), the **staggering** benefits of exercise become clear.

So you can see why the Academy of Medical Colleges was going on about it. It is not unreasonable to think that getting active will make you biologically younger. The evidence suggests that is exactly what happens. So when my friend Marion said that she would like to slice a year off her age when her birthday came round, she was not far off the possible. You cannot stop ageing, but you can slow it down.

WHY GETTING MORE ACTIVE REALLY IS FITNESS FRIENDLY:

✓ It boosts your well-being straight away.

✓ It improves your fitness measurably over a few weeks.

✓ It dramatically reduces the risk of heart disease, stroke, dementia and some cancers, and helps prevent type 2 diabetes and depression.

✓ It helps you keep healthy even with medical conditions.

And as we shall see, getting fitter is about getting back in control of your health as your fitness gap begins to close. We can prevent many things that are harmful to our health, but we need to accept that we can't prevent everything, and hope for a bit of luck to avoid what we can't prevent. But we know that improving our physical well-being helps our mental resilience too, so we are in a better position to manage unwelcome events if they come (see also Chapter 6).

What activities help?

The short answer is 'almost anything you can think of' – every little bit of activity counts. What works best is what you enjoy doing so you keep doing it. And something that stretches you just a bit further than your comfort zone will maximise the energy you spend and the resilience you build.

ACTIVITIES TO GET YOU GOING

You choose. Have you tried ...

✓ yoga?

✓ running round the block once – then twice, then three times ... ?

✓ walking briskly, with a friend?

✓ Zumba, or a stretch and fitness class at your local gym or community centre?

✓ swimming – a great way to keep active and limbered up.

What does fitness look like?

Being fitter can make you feel better, and it shows, not just in your face but in everything you do. You will have a combination of energy, strength and ease of movement. Your posture will be stable and upright whether you're sitting, standing or moving. Your body will be more resilient and your mind motivated and alert for what you want to do. Have a go at Pearl No. 3: The Plumb Line.

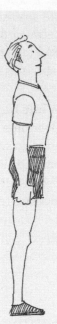

PEARL NO. 3: THE PLUMB LINE

Don't be a tortoise ... be a plumb line.

✓ **Stand up** as straight, tall and erect as you can.

✓ **Head up** and back, and chin tucked in a little, as if a plumb line was attached from the ceiling to the top of the back of your head. It stops you being a tortoise.

✓ **Shoulders relaxed.**

✓ **Tummy pulled in.**

✓ **Legs ready to swing** from the hips and

✓ **arms swinging – sometimes**, but it depends what else you're doing.

Posture is priceless: try to practise this posture whenever you're walking or standing.

Let's look at the five features of fitness that work together to provide this combination. In reality they overlap and many of the ordinary and enjoyable activities you do will provide some of each. Here they are, all starting (or sort of) with an 'S':

1. **Stamina** (your cardiovascular powerhouse).
2. **Strength** (essential for your muscle power, endurance and metabolic health).
3. **Suppleness** (essential so your muscles and joints don't stiffen, snap or rub).
4. **Skills** (posture, balance and coordination).
5. **pSychology** (boosts mental well-being **and** uses your own mental resources).

In fact, there are two more ingredients of physical fitness and they both begin with 'S' too. The first is Substance (see Chapter 4) and the second is Sleep (see Chapter 3).

A rough guide to your fitness now

Your resting pulse rate is a simple guide to your physical fitness. Unless you are on medication, have a fever or a thyroid problem not yet under control, are anxious or on your third cup of coffee, your pulse will be somewhere between 60–100, with 70–80 being the range for most adults who aren't athletes. In general, the lower your pulse the fitter you are. NHS Choices (www.nhs.uk) has a good section on pulse rate fitness.

What happens when you start getting active

Over time as you get fitter your pulse rate is likely to become a bit slower, and you will be able to do more intense activity before you get breathless or tired. Eventually, your resting blood pressure will become lower too. But DURING EXERCISE your pulse, breathing rate and blood pressure will increase temporarily.

You are working your heart harder to stretch its capacity, pumping power and efficiency, which boosts your cardiovascular fitness. If you have just had a heart attack or a significant heart problem, please seek advice before you increase your activity.

Setting fitness free: transforming the ordinary into the extraordinary

The plan is that every day you'll do something towards increasing your stamina, strength, suppleness and skills. Your own personal psychology will help and be helped in return. Remember that every bit of activity counts and it's rarely too late to start or too soon to get going.

Stamina: the heart of fitness
Staying power

The word stamina applies equally well to your ability to sustain prolonged physical *or* mental activity. The more we discover how activity improves our physical stamina the more we find it helps our mind and mood as well (see also Chapter 3).

Activities like brisk walking, swimming, cycling, dancing and playing tennis, all increase your pulse and breathing rate and help to boost your heart and stimulate your circulation. Moderately intense activity makes you breathless but still just able to talk. Intense activity makes you too breathless to talk. In fact, lots of 'ordinary' activities do this too, like gardening or active housework.

Dynamic activities are referred to as 'cardiovascular' exercise because of the benefits they bring to the heart and circulation. But that's not all they do. They keep your metabolic system healthy, improve your brain function, build strength in the muscles you actively use and maintain their suppleness and skill.

Dynamic activity, where your whole body is on the move, is mostly 'aerobic'. This means you use more oxygen during the activity itself and get more breathless as your lungs are stimulated to take more in, but your breathing rate and pulse return to normal fairly soon afterwards.

Lungs on legs

Even **2 minutes** of exercise done regularly each week can make a difference. Both regular chunks and lots of little bits of exercise work well to build stamina. Anything is better than nothing, and every little bit counts.

The recommendation for adults is do a minimum of 30 minutes of moderately intense activity at least 5 days per week – or about 150 minutes in total. But you don't have to do it all at once. You can spread your 'daily dose' throughout the day, and your total throughout the week.

Working up bit by bit

If you've been inactive, it's good to work up to your target gradually. Start with mild activity, such as walking at ordinary speed (which will only make you breathless if you're very unfit), and increase over four weeks to moderate activity such as brisk walking or jogging (which will start to get you fitter). Move to more intense activity over the next two to four months if you can, such as walking briskly uphill (great for bone strength), running, or rowing on the machine at the gym.

The joy of walking

Walking at a leisurely pace shouldn't make you breathless. But it can be enjoyable and it's a great way to start exercising. You get fresh air, limber up and can practise your plumb line posture (see Pearl No. 3 on page 26) and balance. Even leisurely walking will stretch and activate your leg muscles, particularly in your trunk, hips, thighs and calves, and on a sunny day will help you produce a bit more vitamin D.

But from the point of view of 'stamina', if your walking *remains* leisurely you probably won't build up your stamina or increase your fitness much.

You can help it build up stamina simply by increasing your speed. You get more breathless as you start to push your heart, circulation and leg muscles, because you need lots more oxygen to do this. Boost your rhythm and speed even more with Nordic walking using two hiking sticks or join a rambling club. Just step outside your front door and get going – all you need is a pair of comfy shoes and your front door key.

Or try getting off the bus a stop earlier or park further away, and walk briskly to your destination. This way you can clock up some of your moderately intense activity in the routine journeys you make.

One of the long-term benefits of increasing your stamina is that you can do more demanding exercise for longer before you start to get uncomfortably breathless, rather than panting with the slightest exertion, like when you're unfit.

Strength: more power to your elbow

Strength is the force generated by muscles working to overcome a resistance. A resistance could be the weight of something you lift or the resistance of an elastic band you stretch. This is the basis of key strengthening exercise to get fitter and stay fitter. You want to maintain strength to look after yourself when you're older and get out of a chair unassisted. Lay the groundwork now, in your 60s, to be stronger in your 70s and beyond.

What strength does for you

Over time, exercising against resistance makes you stronger and improves your energy, metabolism, well-being, resilience and joie de vivre too.

Muscle strength is critical for preventing falls (so reduces the risk of fractures), as powerful muscles can more rapidly correct a wobble before you hit the floor. And this, in turn, protects your head from impact injuries, saving a lot of brain cells!

Muscle-strengthening exercises builds bone strength so they are less likely to fracture if you do fall. This is particularly important for women after menopause, when bones and muscles lose strength more quickly. And if you have weaker bones already (osteopenia or osteoporosis, see Chapter 5) then muscle strengthening exercises and good brisk walking are great ways of building up your bone-strength.

Last but not least, stronger muscles stabilise joints making them more efficient, and can help you sustain your cardiovascular activity better.

'Tired all the time'

When you are unfit you tire very easily, and this is a very common complaint that takes people to their GP (see Chapter 4). It is important to take this problem seriously if it's unusual for you to feel like this. Occasionally there is a physical problem, for example anaemia or an underactive thyroid, or you may be depressed. If you are tired all the time these possibilities need to be ruled out. But, more often than not, there is no single thing 'wrong' and the real problem is simply that you are out of condition.

This DOESN'T mean that 'it doesn't matter'. It means that it matters VERY MUCH. It's a warning sign to get fitter and back in condition before your fitness gap widens even more through inactivity, when you feel you 'haven't got the energy' to get going. Strengthening your muscles is a very important part of getting this energy back and feeling, as well as being, fitter.

Some technical stuff and mixing strength and stamina

There are two aspects to muscle strength. Firstly, there is the maximum strength a muscle/s can exert during a single action. Secondly, there is the maximum number of continuous repetitions of muscle action possible, over a single exercise session, before it tires. This is muscular endurance.

Cardiovascular exercise for stamina is primarily 'aerobic' work (oxygen using) and is often contrasted with single action strengthening exercise and the early phase of muscular endurance exercise, which is more 'anaerobic' work (oxygen isn't used straight away).

But continuously repeating muscle activity against resistance (the later phase of endurance) starts to use up extra oxygen during the exercise itself, and overall it becomes a mix of aerobic and anaerobic work. So endurance links in and overlaps with stamina. But the component of anaerobic work boosts the need for extra oxygen for several hours afterwards. This means it helps you burn up extra calories even **after** the exercise itself has finished (increasing your resting metabolic rate, see Chapter 4) - an added bonus if you're trying to lose weight.

So, when you go for a steady jog or brisk walk, take your resistance band (see below) with you and stop en route to do a minute or two upper limb strengthening exercise (see page 37), or do two minutes of strengthening when you get back home if that's easier.

Using weights and resistance bands to improve muscle strength

If you use simple weights or a resistance band regularly, to exercise muscle groups, you will gradually increase their strength. Over time you will be able to lift heavier objects as you build up to a new level of comfortable, maximum muscle strength. You may notice your muscles are firmer and more toned up – visible evidence of your increasing fitness.

To maintain your stamina and build your strength your muscles and joints need to remain supple and flexible rather than stiff and tight. They also need to be well coordinated and their movements balanced and controlled. This brings us straight to the next two features of fitness, suppleness and skill.

Suppleness: the 'ease' of it
Suppleness is flexibility

Suppleness is the ease with which a joint moves through its full range. It is not floppiness and depends on appropriate muscle tone during rest or activity.

'Stiffness' is the opposite of suppleness and is one of the most common complaints of ageing. As we get older, we get stiffer more quickly with inactivity, but it can affect us well before our 60s if we're used to sitting for a long time. It is particularly troublesome for women as the structure of connective tissue changes after the menopause making it less elastic (see Chapter 5). Joint surfaces need to be smooth and well lubricated to glide easily over each other.

Preventing stiffness and maintaining suppleness

Do this simple stretching exercise for your lower limbs now (there are more later in the chapter):

Stand with your legs a shoulder width apart, resting your hands against a wall or a tabletop for stability. Gently bend at your hips and knees until you feel the stretching in your legs and hold to a count of ten. Lift yourself an inch or two, then lower yourself again – repeat this ten times. It's a good exercise to do when you've been sitting down too long.

TOP TIPS TO AVOID STIFFNESS AND MAINTAIN SUPPLENESS

✓ **Don't stay still for too long.** If you are sitting at work or reading, set an alarm to remind you to get up and stretch (see above) for 1–2 minutes every 20 minutes. It helps.

✓ **Don't overdo it.** At the other end of the spectrum, don't bring unintended stiffness on yourself by unthinking overuse. This can happen with *over-aggressive* repetition, which causes inflammation.

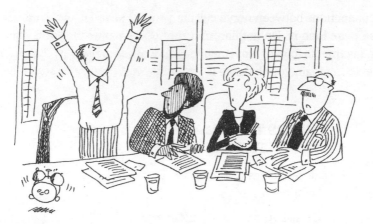

It's time to look at posture, balance and coordination. Maintaining an upright posture is one of the most important features of fitness. It brings us to your balance and movement skills.

Skill: the control of it

Don't fall over

The whole point of balance and coordination is to keep you **upright, mobile and safe from falling**. So the first thing you need is to be awake and alert.

Your brain will use all the information it can get to keep you in the upright position. Your vision, hearing, personal gyroscopes (the balance organs deep in your ears), the sensations from your muscles and joints and even the skin of your feet are **all** used in the mix of what helps to keep you upright and in control of your position in space.

When any one or more of these important sources of information are unavailable or impaired, the brain will be at a disadvantage, and you will need to compensate for the loss if you can. And, of course, if your brain itself is not working well – for example, if you've had a stroke – then you will need expert help and lots of practice to recover the capacity to remain upright and move about.

Baby steps

We often forget that a long time ago, we **did** have to learn to pull ourselves upright and walk. Most of us crawled before we could toddle. In fact, standing upright, walking and turning are all learned skills.

Most of the time your brain controls your learned movements without you realising what's happening. But if you don't keep active you start to lose the connections between nerve cells in your brain and spinal cord – it really is **use it or lose it**. Do nothing, and the special nerve networks controlling fine adjustments to your movement do not work as efficiently, so you become less able to regain your balance if you move quickly, turn or stumble.

THINGS THAT MAKE YOU GO BUMP IN THE NIGHT (AND DAY)

Here are a dozen things that make you unsteady, six for the feet and legs, and six for the rest of you:

The leg destabilisers:

1. foot pain, whatever the cause

2. inappropriate shoes (high-heeled or ill-fitting)

3. uncut toenails

4. loss of sensation in the feet, whatever the cause

5. joint stiffness and pain in the spine and legs

6. muscle weakness, especially in the trunk and legs

The system destabilisers:

1. poor vision

2. poor balance mechanisms

3. excess weight

4. poor diet

5. an excess of alcohol

6. MPs (Medicine Prescribed by your GP. Seek advice if they're causing dizziness)

You could add to the list. But the important thing, as always, is what can be done. Many hazards are lifestyle related and can be removed, reduced or managed, as we will see in Chapter 5. Just think of every aspect of getting fitter, including improving your balance and posture, as a win-win activity. At the end of this chapter we'll reflect on the psychology of activity, what you get from getting active and how your psychology, in its turn, can transform your good intentions into action. But right now … **it's rehearsal time.**

'Triple S' exercises for strength, suppleness and skill

On your marks …

This is a taste of what's coming up. Do each one daily, or as often as you can.

- **Neck flexibility and posture**: to avoid stiffness.
- **Shoulder, upper limb and chest muscle flexibility**: the upper limb girdle.
- **Shoulder, upper limb and chest muscle strengthening**: the upper limb girdle again.
- **Spinal strength, stability and flexibility**: for your 'core' muscles.
- **Hip flexibility**.
- **Hip strength**.
- **Knee strengthening**: three times daily for weak knees, otherwise daily if you can.
- **Knee flexibility**: if you can.
- **Flexibility and stretchiness** of muscles at the back of the lower limbs.
- **Leg and foot strengthening**.
- **Balance and coordination skills**.

Putting it all together

Think about getting into a routine of doing **10 minutes** of basic strength, suppleness and skill exercises every day. Decide where and when you're going to do them. You can't do everything on the list in 10 minutes – but do at least four 'suppleness', one 'skill' and one upper and lower limb strengthening exercise every day. You will ring the changes with the strengthening exercises. Do the core muscle exercises at least three times a week. It helps to remember that brisk walking and good posture also help build 'core' and lower-limb strength.

A suggested routine is: start with suppleness, move to strength and finish with skill. Stop an exercise if it's painful. And always remember your posture – stand up straight, don't be a tortoise (see page 26). With practice, you can extend your exercises to keep on getting fitter.

Use the rest of the day as well. You can stretch and flex standing in queues, watching the news and waiting for the kettle to boil. If you feel bored, keep a sudoku or crossword somewhere on the wall. Aim to crack it while you're stretching.

What you'll need

You will need two bought or homemade dumb-bells (1–3kg to start) and a resistance band with an appropriate stretch. The shorter the length of band between your hands the harder it will be to stretch. A longer length between your hands will be easier to stretch to reach the desired length. Resistance bands usually come with an accompanying booklet of exercises, and may show which ones can be done sitting down – useful if you are in a wheelchair. You can get these online, or from big supermarkets with a fitness section.

Look before you leap

Before you exercise, ensure you're safe. Check there are no slippery mats or water spills around and that you've got a clear area in which to spread your arms.

If underlying health issues might be affected by exercising, ask for medical advice beforehand.

When you start, take breaks and don't overstrain your muscles

It is important not to lift a weight that's too heavy. If you do, you run the risk of over-stretching or even tearing your muscle. This is a painful injury and it takes time to recover. It may put you out of action for a few weeks, something to be avoided if you can.

Preventing overstrain is why most strengthening exercises have a recommended number of repeats. You should rest after the recommended number, and work to increase it gradually if needed, to avoid going overboard.

But you must remember that if you haven't been active for years, you are bound to have bit of aching and stiffness a day or so after exercising, as your muscles gradually adapt to being used more. This is sometimes called delayed onset muscle soreness (DOMS). Please don't be put off when it happens.

Get set ...

Leaping into activity without warning is occasionally required in real life. Without it we couldn't escape danger, or run for the bus, for example.

Some people choose to do warm-up exercises prior to more intense activity, although you don't need to do warm-ups before walking, for example, just start walking at a gentle pace and gradually increase your speed until you're walking as briskly as you can. However, if you have tight hamstrings and calves you will feel more comfortable if you do some stretching exercises first.

Go!
Neck flexibility and posture

Neck stiffness is a common problem. Look around you – how many people are stooped over mobile phones at bus stops, or slumped over a laptop at work? Without a supple neck you can't look left and right to cross the road, or turn your head when you're driving a car. It is important to do neck suppleness exercises daily. Try these:

- Stand in a relaxed but erect posture.
- Rotate your head to the left and look as far as you can over your left shoulder.
- Bring your head gently back to the midline again.
- Repeat this five times, each time stretching back to look over your shoulder.
- Don't force the rotation if it's painful, stop before that happens.
- Then repeat to the other side.

When you do this, don't do big circles of your head on your neck, stick to half rotations.

Poor posture due to weak neck muscles can tend to thrust your head forward. This leads to gradual loss of the natural curve of the neck, which is convex forwards and keeps your head back and your eyes looking straight ahead rather than downwards. You end up looking at the ground. So posture is important, and you need to remind yourself about it continually. It's worth revisiting Pearl No. 3 (see page 26), concentrating on pulling the back of your head up and back, and stand up tall like you're being pulled on a piece of string from the top of your head – resisting the forward thrusting tendency of your head.

Your shoulders and their girdle: full girdle flexibility

You have upper (shoulder) and lower (hip) limb girdles. Your upper girdle, comprising your shoulder and collar bones, is built for incredible multi-directional mobility of your shoulders, which get stiff if they're not used. The following exercise, known as the backwards butterfly, is more challenging than it looks. If you have persistent pain and stiffness of the shoulder (frozen shoulder), you may not be able to do it immediately. You could do it gently on the side that is unaffected – but don't force it on the painful side – wait till you're ready and check with your GP. You may already have seen a physiotherapist – if so, follow the advice given to you.

Your movements should be slow, gentle and very controlled. You may find that doing one shoulder at a time is better to begin with. The tendency is to bring the arms round again before they have brushed past your ears. But the goal is to reach further back than that in a very controlled way – not whizzing your arms round as if they were windmills.

- Stand with your arms in a loose, relaxed position, palms forward.
- Lift one or both outstretched arms up in front of you. Continue to lift your outstretched arm(s) up and backwards, brushing your ear(s) as they pass behind your head.
- As you reach the limit of backwards stretch your arm(s) will automatically be guided downwards and outwards.
- Gently bring them back to the starting position.
- Repeat. If you started with one shoulder and the other is not painful, do five gentle revolutions on the left and five on the right.

For undoing hunched shoulders:

- Pull your shoulders back, with your hands clasped behind you, so your shoulder blades come together more closely. It will push your chest out a bit.
- Hold the position for about five seconds, relax for five seconds, and repeat five times.

You will feel the muscles being pulled together tightly and then relaxing. It's usually a nice feeling, and you can do it anytime, anywhere. A lot of muscle tension can creep into hunched shoulders, especially if you sit stooped at a desk for hours.

Strengthening your upper limbs, chest and shoulders: the full girdle, again

Your upper limbs and their girdle need regular strengthening so that all the muscles are strong and stable. They 'brace' your shoulders, strengthen your chest muscles and build the lifting and pushing power of your arms.

The best way of strengthening your upper limb girdle and your arms is a good old 'chest expansion', and uses your resistance band:

- Stand tall and erect with your shoulders relaxed.
- Hold your resistance band with each hand so you have about half its length between your hands.
- Slowly and gently stretch the band out as you fully extend your arms.
- If you cannot extend your arms to their full span, increase the length of band between your hands.
- Hold the position for a second or two and then very slowly relax the band to its resting state. Repeat five times.

For exercising your upper limbs – biceps, wrist muscles and hand muscles – it is useful to have two dumb-bells, or homemade weights (bags of rice, for example). Start by lifting the dumb-bells from waist height to shoulder height, exercising each arm at a time. After a week or two, lift weights with both arms simultaneously, again to shoulder height:

- Stand or sit erect but relaxed.
- Start with 1kg weight and grip it with one hand.
- Lift the weight over 3–5 seconds to shoulder height, flexing at the elbow.
- Repeat cycles with smooth, controlled arcs of movement five times on each arm.

Note: depending on the resting position of your hands you will exercise a slightly different set of wrist-lifting muscles. If your palms face forwards as you grip the weight, you will be using wrist 'flexors'. If you start with your palms facing your side, you will be using your 'drinking-mug muscles'. If you start with your palm facing backwards you will use your wrist 'extensors'. Check which is easiest for you and avoid any painful movement.

After about four weeks, depending on your ability and prior fitness experience, you can extend the exercise to involve additional muscles. You can start to lift the weights above shoulder height, but still with some bend at the elbow: you will use additional shoulder muscles to elevate your loaded arm.

You could extend the exercise even further over the next 2–4 weeks working towards holding the weights with fully outstretched arms above your head. As you do so you move your whole upper limb girdle on your upper back, using your powerful back muscles.

For exercising your triceps and your shoulder muscles a resistance band is essential:

- Stand in a relaxed position.
- Dangle the band vertically downwards over the back of your right shoulder with your right hand about halfway down the band.
- Bring your left arm back behind you, elbow bent and forearm horizontal, so your left hand can touch the tip of your right shoulder blade.
- Grasp the dangling resistance band with your left hand so you have about half its length between your two hands: a quarter length dangling from each hand.
- Keep your left forearm horizontal and check the tension in the band between your hands.

- Gently extend your right arm upwards straightening the elbow, so it is fully outstretched. Hold the position for five seconds if you can then relax the band slowly to its start position.
- Repeat five times each side, if you can.
- If it is too difficult to stretch the band fully, extend your arms so there is a longer length between your hands and less stretch is needed.

To strengthen your grip, use an old tennis ball. The following exercise strengthens the tiny muscles in your hand, but also the forearm muscles, which stabilise your wrist and bend your fingers into a grip position. Before and after this exercise, stretch your fingers and thumbs out wide on both hands and hold the position for 5 seconds. Relax them completely and repeat five times. Then do your hand squeezes.

Stand or sit in a relaxed position, and exercise one hand at a time:

- Stretch your left arm full length in front of you, holding the tennis ball in your left hand.
- Curl the fingers and thumb of your left hand around the ball, and squeeze as firmly as you comfortably can. Hold the position for 5 seconds. Relax the grip – but keep your fingers and thumb flexed round the ball so you don't drop it. Repeat ten times.
- Then relax your left hand and arm, and transfer the ball to your right hand. Repeat the exercise with your right hand, with your right arm outstretched.

Carry the tennis ball around with you, and exercise your grip if you feel tension building up so you avoid squeezing your jaw muscles.

An alternative to a ball is a hand-grip for building your grip strength. These are sprung metal hinges with foam-covered handles (a bit like spring-loaded nut-crackers). They are cheap in fitness shops or online.

Spinal strength and stability: building your 'core' muscles
Your core muscles provide protection for your abdominal organs and support for your spine and hip girdle. Walking helps your core muscles too. Every time you walk briskly, especially with a good posture, you'll be exercising your core. When you practise mindful breathing (see Chapter 3) you'll be aware how much breathing itself is a core strengthening exercise.

Almost everything you do when you lean over, pick things up or twist and shout involves bracing your core abdominal and lower back muscles.

Building core muscle strength can help you prevent and manage back pain, one of the commonest complaints at any age. Strengthening the muscles of your abdominal wall also makes them more resistant to developing hernias. You can also develop a toned body shape too.

Perhaps the most well-known and widely used core exercise is the 'sit-up', which uses your core muscles, hip flexors and back muscles too.

The exercise shown here is not a full sit-up (there are many examples of this on the internet), but a simple and very 'do-able' core strengthening and stability routine. But for ringing the changes please do look on the web or think of going to a fitness class, where a trainer can advise if needed.

If you have a hernia or back problems, please ask your GP what is safe to do first.

- Lie down, with your hands behind your head.
- Lift your right leg about 12 inches off the ground and hold it there for 10 seconds.
- Lower it slowly. Then repeat with your left leg. Repeat this five times for each leg.
- Then lift both legs together about 12 inches off the ground.
- Criss-cross your feet ten times.
- Lower both feet slowly to the ground.

You may need to work up to the 'both legs together' bit gradually, over about four weeks, starting with lifting your legs together and holding them for 5–10 seconds in the air, before lowering them slowly again. Build up to criss-crossing them, from two to ten times, over a further four weeks.

Hip and thigh flexibility

Your hips are ball and socket joints made by the ball of your thighbone in the socket of your pelvis. Your hip joint can bend up at the front, stretch back, move out to the side and swing across to your other side. The thighbone can twist and rotate inwards and outwards, which makes the toes and knee face inwards and outwards too.

These two simple exercises help to keep the soft tissues around the hip joint supple so that twisting your hip outwards or bringing your thigh across to the other side are as flexible as possible. If you've had a hip replacement, check when these are safe for you to do.

For keeping your hips and thighs flexible:

- Lie on your back on the floor.
- Flex your left knee up, keeping your left foot flat on the floor.
- Flex your right knee up and let your right leg fall outwards at the hip.

- Raise your right foot and bring your right ankle to rest against your flexed left knee.
- Very, very gently bounce your right bent knee with your right hand. **Don't force it.** If it's painful don't bounce it, hold for a few seconds and repeat on the other side.

Do five each side if you can, but **none at all** if it's painful. If it's stiff but possible, work up gradually.

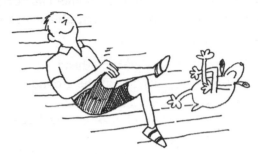

For keeping your hips and thighs supple:

- Lie on the floor with both legs straight.
- Flex up your right knee. Put your right foot on the floor on the far side of your left knee.
- Hold it there for 5 seconds, then stretch your right leg out straight on the floor again.
- Repeat this five times, then …
- … do it on the other side.

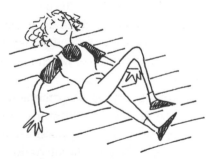

Hip strengthening exercises
Please check with your GP or physiotherapist if you've just had hip joint replacement surgery. Don't do 'sit-to-stands' from low down until advised it's OK to do.

The key exercise for your hips is called the 'sit-to-stand':

- Sit on a chair without armrests (yes, do sit, but not for long …).
- Without using your hands, stand up and sit down again in a single movement and repeat ten times. If that's too easy, do 20 and gradually work up to 30 in one minute.
- Yes – the cycle of repeats should be completed within ONE MINUTE.

Repeated 'sit-to-stands' **can predict future fitness,** well-being and longevity. If you're female and can do, on average, 35 'sit-to-stands' in one minute or 37 if you're male, that predicts greater robustness for the future. Being able to move quickly and stably from sitting to standing is one of the KEY things you need to be able to do to keep independent when you get older. It requires strong hip muscles, but also good coordination and balance control of your trunk.

If that's too easy then sit on something lower than the position of your bent knee (like the bottom step of your stairs, or a low stool) and do the same routine. When your bottom is lower than your hip you have to use more energy to stand up.

Knee strengthening: the quads

Your quads (short for quadriceps, because this huge muscle has four sections) are important postural muscles and among the strongest in your body. They need to be because they keep your legs straight and you upright. They form the sturdy columns on which your whole body pivots on the ground each time you take a step.

To strengthen your quads, try the following exercise:

- Sit down (again).
- Extend you left leg with the knee straight: you use your quads for this.
- Tighten your quads (muscles at the front and sides of your thigh) **HARD.**
- Hold this position for 30 seconds: count them.
- Then relax that leg, and immediately repeat with the other leg.
- Hold the other leg as before, with the **QUADS HARD**, count to 30, then relax.
- Repeat the sequence five times with each leg in turn: 5 minutes total time.

These are **KEY EXERCISES** for strengthening the knee, including during recovery from an acute knee injury. If you have a knee problem, it's a good idea to do your quad exercises more intensively: 5 minutes three times daily minimum – you can do it whenever you're sitting down.

Knee flexibility: squats

If you have painful or very weak knees then it may be too uncomfortable to squat because it puts your weight on your flexed knee joints. If they are inflamed it will be painful. If so, it may be better to concentrate first on strengthening your knees with your QEs. So, avoid squatting if you have a very acute (recent) knee problem.

If your knees are not painful, gentle squats are good for the flexibility of soft tissues around them. First, check that you can bend up each knee in turn before you do weight-bearing squats. If you can bend them easily try the following knee squats gently, these will help flexibility:

- Stand with your feet apart (a shoulder's width).
- Bending at your hips and knees, touch the floor between your knees with your fingertips, keeping your back as straight as possible (100 per cent is impossible).
- If you can, put your palms flat down on the floor. Work up to this gradually if you can't do it straight away.
- Repeat ten times, as smoothly as you can, then stop.

Over time, if you can do this without discomfort, slightly increase the distance between your feet checking each time that you are stable.

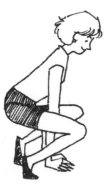

Stretching and strengthening the muscles at the back of your lower limbs

If you have recently hurt your back or suffer from low back pain, check with your physiotherapist or GP if these are OK for you. Go gently, and stop if it is painful.

The 'hamstrings' above the knee and the calf muscles below it are also strong postural muscles, which keep you upright. If they get tight, it is more difficult and sometimes painful to walk or run. Wearing high heels makes the calf muscles tighter: avoid them if possible. Stretching them regularly helps. Try the following exercise:

- Keeping your back straight, gently bend forward at the hips, until your back itself is horizontal (but with its natural curve). You should feel your hamstrings (at the back of your thighs) stretching.
- If you can, hold the position for 10 seconds, then relax and stand up.
- Repeat five times.

You could extend the exercise and stretch your hamstrings more by curling your back forward to touch your toes. But you should NOT do this if you have back problems or sciatica, or if you find it hurts.

It is also important to stretch your calf muscles. Try the following:

- Hold on to a rail or counter.
- Bend one knee to shorten your height.
- Hold the other leg straight, stretching it back from your extended hip.
- Check that the ball of your foot on the extended leg is flat on the floor with the heel slightly raised. You will feel your hams and your calves being stretched.
- Hold that stretch, gently and rhythmically shifting your weight up and down on the ball of that foot for 30 seconds.
- Switch to the other leg, and repeat.
- Do five each side, if you can.

If you have a long-distance drive, plan frequent stops to get out and stretch your calves and hamstrings. Then flex each hip up, one at a time, clasping your flexed knee to your chest, and repeat a few times each side. Then stretch your whole spine by pulling yourself as tall as you can. With each arm in turn, reaching up to the sky, pointing your index finger as high as you can.

Exercises for strong, stable legs, feet and toes

The bulky calf muscles at the back of your lower legs fit into your Achilles tendon at the back of your heels. These are some of the strongest tendons you have. You exercise your calves when you stand on tiptoe. Other calf muscles, and muscles at the sides and front of your leg, send tendons into your feet to move your toes.

Standing on tiptoes is so simple that you can do it anywhere: standing in a queue, looking out at the view or while doing something that you do each day. Do it waiting for the kettle to boil! If you're a bit wobbly – hold on to a tabletop or chair or put your hand against the wall – and go for it. Stand on your tiptoes for three minutes, tall as you can.

For even more calf muscle strength try the following:

- Find a low step. (Don't use a stool – it might tip up. When you do it on the flat, your calves don't work as hard as they do with a step.)
- Put the front half of your left foot on the lowest step you have, so your heel is 'hanging'.
- Hold on to something secure with one hand, the wall usually, and gently rise up and down five–ten times.
- Repeat with the other foot.
- If you feel unsteady at any time – put both feet down immediately.

Before you get out of bed in the morning, loosen the stiffness that builds up in your feet and ankles overnight. Screw up your toes – then spread them out and wriggle them thoroughly. Then rotate your ankles outwards for half a minute. Then flex your ankles bringing your feet up towards you – stretching your calves gently. Then relax them, and point your feet down like a ballet dancer. Do that several times, and finish off with some ankle rotations again. If you get cramp in your toes – pull the front of your foot towards your leg for a few seconds.

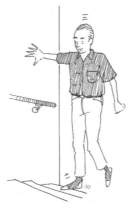

Better balance

Balance is important, and checking it regularly will help you avoid problems further down the line. The ability to stand on one leg, for example, is a good predictor of future brain health (see also Chapter 4). Here are a few suggested exercises. If you can do them, that's marvellous, keep it up. If you can't do them at all, it suggests that you might have a balance problem and you should chat to your GP about it fairly soon.

First, please check the floor isn't slippery, and don't do these if you've been drinking alcohol within the last 4 hours:

- Stand on one leg with your eyes open and raise the other, holding it in the air for 30 seconds, if you can.
- Try it on the other leg.
- Can you get to one minute on each leg before feeling unsteady and putting your raised foot down again?
- If so, then try to rotate your raised foot while you stand on the other leg. See if you can build up to a minute on each leg while rotating the other foot.

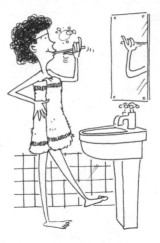

One day, try it with your raised leg flexed at the hip and knee: so you can hug your raised leg. Is it easier or more difficult?

After a week or two, try it with your eyes shut … BUT ONLY if you're in a safe place and not on a slippery floor. And OPEN YOUR EYES IMMEDIATELY if you feel unsteady.

None of us like toeing the line, but in this case it's useful. Draw an imaginary (or real) line on the floor. Take off your shoes and walk 'heel to toe' along the line. Try to walk across the room, turn round, and come back again. Keep your arms outstretched if you want.

If you can't do it because you wobble too much, increase the distance between your heel and your toe by about 6 inches and try that. Then see if you can work up to a strict 'heel to toe' over a few weeks.

Mixing and matching ... again

You can do all the exercises described above at home with minimal equipment – and they're a great start to keep you ticking along. But if you're looking for variety, or keen to get out of the house as well, there is evidence that mixing an exercise class once a week with your daily home exercises is a very good combo, and better than either on their own.

Pilates is excellent for core muscle strength, balance and coordination. And T'ai Chi is great for lower limb muscle and bone strength and for balance. It is particularly good for women if kept up in the long term.

Cycling clubs and running clubs are springing up all over the country (parkrun is particularly good) and there are many walking and rambling clubs. Your local leisure centre or gym is bound to run classes, or maybe someone runs a yoga, Pilates or Zumba session in your village or local hall? Go and have a sample session, or check out their timetables online – take a friend along if you're feeling shy.

If you're already a member of a social or games club like bridge, bowls or bingo for instance, then fantastic, good for you. Why not expand its fun and fitness element a bit? You could club together for a Pilates or yoga teacher to come by, or spend five minutes doing simple stretches and strengthening exercises before you start your main game each week.

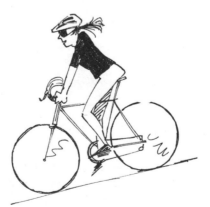

Resolutions, routines and blowing it

Q: What to do if you've only got 2 minutes?
A: Stretch as much as you can, and strengthen your upper limbs. For everything else walk, walk and walk some more, whenever you can.

WHAT TO DO WHEN IT ALL GOES PEAR SHAPED:

✓ **It's all gone out of the window** and you've not done anything active all week – don't beat yourself up, just start again. Try asking yourself why you stopped. Has it been difficult to get a routine going at all? The next section may help. It may also help to join an exercise class once a week, it may be enjoyable and motivate you to do just a little bit on your own as well.

✓ **It's all too much** – OK, cherry pick. Is there something that hurts each time you try it? Do you need to sort out why? Have a think what it might be: a recent injury, your medical history, arthritis perhaps? Check it out if it's 'new to you' and persists.

✓ **Praise yourself** – find one small thing to praise yourself for – even if it's just the question you asked yourself about why you haven't managed to keep going. Beating yourself up doesn't work. Try to sort whatever the problem is. Are you trying at the wrong time of the day? Just do your best.

The pSychology of getting active

You feel better, think better and do better

Knowledge on its own is rarely enough to actually change your fitness-finding behaviour. You need to change your behaviour effectively, and not only get started but keep going. You don't need to be a psychologist to make constructive change in your life BUT ... it can help to use some tools of the trade.

The psychology of change
Some SMART tips

We didn't invent these. SMART approaches to implementing changes in life are widely used in the workplace so you may be familiar with them already – they can be hijacked to help make changes that improve your health and well-being. You can harness you own psychology to help you get more active.

In a nutshell, you need to be absolutely clear what your overall objective is, so you can figure out how to achieve it. In fact your goal to get more active has three phases:

1. **starting** to get more active
2. **staying** more active, and ...
3. **pushing** up your activity bit by bit with time

You are more likely to succeed with each phase if you have a **SMART** approach rather than a vague 'wish' to get fitter. SMART is:

- **S**pecific
- **M**easurable
- **A**chievable
- **R**ealistic
- **T**imed.

Your plan needs to be **Specific**. It's no good just saying 'I want my muscles to be stronger'. Instead say something like 'I will strengthen my upper limb muscles by doing "X" stretches with my resistance band'.

You need to have feedback on how effective your action is, so it needs to be **Measurable**. Aim for five repeats, for example, but if you can't reach that straight away, you can work towards it.

The target needs to be **Achievable**. If you are very out of condition stretching a band (e.g. to full 'outstretched arms') may be too much to begin with. It is important to fully stretch out your arms, so make it easier with a longer length of band between your hands until it is achievable. If the resistance band is 'too resistant' you may need a more stretchy band initially.

The target you have specified needs to be **Realistic** too. If you have just had an operation you will be recommended to do more gentle exercises or none at all while you recover.

Finally, it makes sense that there is realistic **Time** in which to achieve your goal. This helps motivation and is a prompt to look closely at what you are doing if you're nowhere near achieving your goal in the time you anticipated. You can always review your time frame if it turns out to have been unrealistic. If you aren't making progress, ask yourself 'Why not?'

Starting to get active

The New Year is a great time for resolutions: flag up the next one but why wait until then? Start tomorrow – or even **right now**, with a few stretches to confirm to yourself that today is the first day of the rest of your new life.

Find the right time of day. Could you fit in your 10-minute 'Triple S' routine shortly after you get up? It can make sense to do it before showering and dressing so you feel toned up and ready for the day.

Staying active

It's important to think of your exercise routine as part of your daily pattern. It is essential, like sleep and breakfast. If your daily routine changes because of travelling or holidays then think ahead to how you'll fit it in wherever you are. It's **THAT** important.

Pushing up

Once you have achieved your target and been doing it easily for a few weeks, **congratulate yourself**. When you reset your objective, set the goal a little higher and push up your limit just a tiny bit, using the SMART approach each time. For example, with the strengthening exercise for the upper limbs, you might move up to a slightly more resistant stretch band after 3–4 months. Look back over the last few weeks and see if you could make the next plan work even better for you. This is a life-long enterprise, and it's under your control.

Resolutions

RESOLUTIONS FOR KEEPING ACTIVE

✓ I will make my 10-minute Triple S exercises part of my daily routine.

✓ I will walk as much as I can, as briskly as I can.

✓ I will do four stretching, two strengthening and one skill-based exercise every day.

Try Pearl No. 4, which is an exercise in attentive listening. It will help prepare you for the next chapter.

PEARL NO. 4: HEAR A PIN DROP

You have two whole minutes for the sound of silence. Find the quietest place you can. Check there is no obvious background noise. Turn your mobile off. Stand, sit on a chair, sit crossed-legged on the floor, or squat if your knees can take it for 2 minutes. You need to concentrate attentively. You need to be alert to the slightest sound, so don't lie down unless you have to – you might drift off to sleep.

Listen, for 2 minutes (a whole 120 seconds please). Attend to the silence outside you. Leave your thoughts alone. Strain your ears. Could you hear a pin drop? How quiet is silence? Give it your whole attention for 2 minutes, to find out.

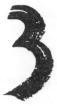

YOUR ATTITUDE AND ITS SOULMATES: YOUR MIND AND MOOD

Plan for happiness and resilience

Happiness is a good thing, not a bad thing

Stuff happens, we can't avoid it (see Chapter 7), but happiness is good, it's not a guilt trip. ***Not being able*** to be happy is an indicator that something is wrong.

So let's embrace happiness, sow seeds for it, nurture it and enjoy it when it comes. It builds resilience, along with all the other things that build fitness, health and well-being. And above all, let's share our happiness, because happiness, like laughter, is infectious.

We need to bust stress when it's harmful (a little is OK – and goes a long way). We need to remove the poisons and dependencies that spoil and chain us, like smoking, excess alcohol and unnecessary drugs (Chapters 3, 5 and 8). We need to try to limit the damage when stuff comes our way and the way of others (see Chapter 7) because we are all interconnected … no one is an island.

This chapter is about your attitude and its soulmates, mind and mood. They're a willing partnership, all in one with your body.

Ageing isn't the problem

So Sod 60! You didn't wake up on your 60th birthday to find you were a different person. You are still you, and your thoughts and feelings reflect the unique person you are. You define yourself, not your age. You can foster your mental and emotional well-being, just as you can build your physical fitness. And as you do, you enrich your mind and mood and develop your resilience to the ups and downs and stuff that happens in life. What's more, this is true whether you have mental or physical conditions or are lucky enough to have none.

Turning 60 and taking stock

Turning 60 is a real opportunity to take stock of who you are and where you're heading. If you're retiring, are you planning to retire from life or for life? If you're going to embrace life, do you know what matters to you?

If you have a sense of purpose and direction it can make all the difference to your self-esteem and emotional well-being. And if you're trying to figure out how you want to live the rest of your life, then understanding what makes you tick is a good place to start.

Finding your attitude

This chapter focuses on mind and mood. Looking after your body helps you look after them too, but there are additional things that are essential for your mental and emotional well-being. They all fit together and you need to maintain them just as you need to look after your body.

You will have your own understanding of soul. But as you take care of your mind and mood and attend to your reflective as well as your outgoing self, you find your own, unique attitude. It is part of your being and radiates something about who you are.

Ageing and the changes it might bring to your mind and mood

Most of the mental and emotional changes we attribute to age are due to everything else that builds up or happens, including the knock-on effects of illnesses, life events, social circumstances and lifestyle. Ageing has a small effect, but it's tiny compared to other things.

Your working brain is essential for your memory, reasoning, decision making and mood, which is why it's so important to take care of your most vital organ – your brain – as well as the rest of your body (see Chapter 5).

In Chapter 1 we recognised that our cognitive skills do decline very slightly as we age. Our memory may not be so brisk and our mental processing slightly slower. But we can compensate for this (see below) and take active steps to slow the decline, as we have seen already.

It's the reflective balance of our judgement, as well as its logical train and relevance to the matter under consideration that counts. Daniel Kahneman's book *Thinking, Fast and Slow* argues that different kinds of thinking are needed for different kinds of tasks, and this is a useful insight.

Some situations require a quick decision for safety's sake: when you're driving, or at work and responsible for other people's safety as well as your own.

We all make mistakes sometimes. But if we persistently make them, and there have been a number of serious errors with repercussions, it's important to work out why. Tiredness, anxiety, stress and low mood may be explanations – and if these are regular symptoms it would be wise to see your doctor to exclude an underlying problem.

The more significant things that affect memory and mental processing as we age are effects of long-term alcohol excess, brain diseases like stroke and (unusually in our 60s) dementia (we will look at these in Chapter 5), and the best thing we can do is to reduce their risk as far as possible while we are able to.

Bereavement and loss and other life events are increasingly common in our 50s and 60s and beyond, and can affect our mental and emotional life. If we lack resilience and support, they can have serious consequences for our emotional well-being. We know that as we get older we tend to accumulate medical conditions and these, together with social factors such as poor housing, poverty and isolation, can all lead to low mood.

The great majority of people do not get anxious or depressed as they age, but unfortunately depression is still common. It's estimated that about 2 million people in the UK aged 65 or over suffer from it, that's 22 per cent of men and 28 per cent of women.

If we assume there is nothing we can do for our mental well-being as we get older, that is false. There is much we can do. But mental well-being, however achieved, doesn't mean that mental illness never happens – and it's important to pick it up and get help if it does. So … **things do sometimes go pear-shaped and mental illness can occur which we can't always prevent. If you are very distressed, or someone else is sufficiently concerned about you to say so – then please, take those concerns seriously and talk to your doctor.**

You can also refer yourself for talking-based therapy locally, through an NHS venture called IAPT (Improving Access to Psychological Therapies). There are more details on the NHS Choices website (www.nhs.uk) or through your GP.

Find the holistic route to mental well-being

The following seven steps will allow your mind and mood to walk well together:

1. **Keep true to yourself**: being you and becoming yourself.
2. **Keep connected with others**, and generous with your resources.
3. **Keep physically active.**
4. **Keep curious**: keep learning, and loving it.
5. **Bust stress**: practise mindfulness – and other good things.
6. **Keep sleep sound**: perchance to dream.
7. **Keep out of harm's way**.

Let's flag up mindfulness here – you may have heard of it already. It's quite a buzzword and we'll discuss it more below. It helps you focus your whole attention on the moment you're in, just as you did when you listened to the sound of silence in Pearl No. 4 (on page 50). It's a wonderful way to reduce stress.

WHAT DOES BEING TRUE TO YOURSELF MEAN TO *YOU*?

✓ Be true to your values.

✓ Do what you think is right.

✓ Don't be persuaded or pushed into something that conflicts with what matters deeply to you, however well intentioned the attempt.

And there were some interesting provisos too:

✓ Keep your values under review – do they still hold true for you?

✓ Know when you can compromise – so as to give and take.

✓ Know when you can't compromise – because it matters so deeply.

Being true to your values is important but so is reflecting and reviewing one's values to check they still hold true. Reflecting, reviewing and acting accordingly are important skills to develop, they matter to what makes you the person you are.

Constantly being unable to act according to one's deepest values and beliefs, or being prevented from doing so, causes stress and distress and diminishes well-being. But we are individuals in relationships. Both extremes – never making compromises, and always making compromises – are likely to undermine well-being. The key is to work out what really matters. When you know that, you'll be clearer about what you can or cannot negotiate.

Being you

Being true to yourself has to be weighed up in the context of your relationships. You have to work out when it is best to give way, when to negotiate and when someone has to give way to you.

Confidence and feeling in control of the important things in your life are good for well-being and a healthy mind and mood. Putting what you believe into practice may take effort, commitment and all your social, ethical and empathetic skills. And you may need help. But if something matters deeply, it's worth it.

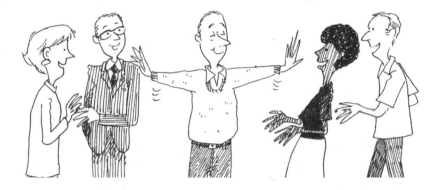

Being you with another, in a close relationship

Sometimes, becoming clearer about what really matters and more confident about acting on it can cause conflict. It becomes apparent that we can no longer go along with other people's expectations or assumptions about us, because they no longer hold true. When people find themselves in that position it can be difficult, particularly if the gulf appears within a close relationship.

A relationship may be valued above all else, and being true to yourself may include the recognition that this is also for you. It is not *necessarily* the existence of difference that prevents relating to someone else, it is what is done with the difference when it exists. We are unique individuals and can only be so if we respect each other's uniqueness too.

And what matters in the close relationship with a partner or spouse is what is shared and how that is valued, as well as what is different.

PEARL NO. 5: FOR A STRONG RELATIONSHIP WITH A PARTNER OR SPOUSE

✓ be yourself with each other

✓ trust each other

✓ listen to each other

✓ share with each other

✓ love each other: not just sex, but that too

✓ forgive each other

✓ learn from the past, and plan for the future

Then, there are rainbows, flowers, foibles, fitness and fears:

✓ laugh with each other

✓ cry with each other

✓ give space to each other

✓ remember each other's special days

✓ accept each other's foibles and failures

✓ help each other thrive

✓ spot each other's red flags: physical and emotional

Keep connected and generous with your resources

Sisterhood, brotherhood, friends, family and beyond

Close relationships and connections with a wider society are all essential to prevent isolation and depression.

Why keep connected? We are social animals and the sense of belonging and love is an important strength to build on. This can include sexual love, but it doesn't have too. It's about relationship, commitment and feeling that we matter to someone and that someone matters to us. These are vital human needs and their absence is a recipe for depression, in our 60s as at any other time. This is at the heart of *why* we need to feel connected.

What connections matter? They all do, potentially. They keep us connected with others and at the same time with ourselves. But it's more than just sharing problems. It's also about building social networks that support us and help us continue to grow.

Not all of us are gregarious and some prefer to be part of a small, familiar network. Most of us have worked this out by the time we hit our 60s. But circumstances can change and the relationships that we once took for granted can ebb away (as we will explore in Chapter 7). So it's worth reminding ourselves now just how important social relationships are.

Pets are great company if you live alone. Having a dog is good exercise (for you) and a good chance to meet others on the end of a lead.

Skype and the internet can help to remain connected with far-flung family and friends. It doesn't replace real, live contact – but it's much better than nothing. Television and radio helps people stay in touch with the wider world too.

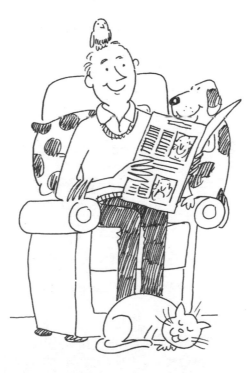

Be generous with your resources

Keeping a generous spirit will help you just as much as others. This can involve small acts of kindness. **Do one good deed a day. Why?** Someone may need what you have to offer, for a start. Why might that be good for your well-being? Because when you really tune into someone else's needs, you exercise your outward thinking. There's no point in giving something if it's not wanted, or might do harm.

You may or may not get anything in return, though it's nice when you receive sincere thanks. But you will always feel the benefit of knowing that, to the best of your ability, you did some small thing for someone else. Even a smile can transform someone else's mood just as it can yours – in an instant. Be generous with your smile where you can.

Using your resources long-term, through activism, working, volunteering and campaigning. If you're on the brink of retirement how are you going to continue to use your resources and experience in the longer term?

You may choose to remain in your current occupation, extending it and taking more responsibility or choose to branch out into a new career. Alternatively, it can be exhilarating to discover new avenues of social involvement. The list is endless: listen to children reading at school, campaign or get involved in local politics, help on your local allotment, run a sports club or a choir, or train to become a mentor and use your resources and experience in a professional setting, helping others reach their potential too.

Whatever you choose, using your resources generously to enrich society can be a wonderful way of keeping connected with others. It usually ends up with exercising your body and stretching your mind too.

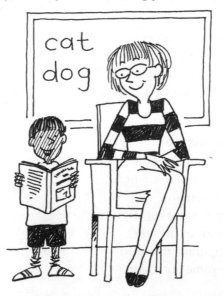

Keeping physically active nurtures your brain, mind and mood

'Mens sana in corpore sano', said the Latin satirist and poet Juvenal, though he based the phrase on a much older text by the Greek philosopher, Thales of Miletus. It means 'a healthy mind in a healthy body' and shows that it is not new news, nor is it rocket science. We saw in the first two chapters that it's not just individual experience and anecdote but plenty of careful research that shows how important physical activity is for improving and maintaining our emotional well-being and thinking skills. And cardiovascular exercise is part of managing both depression and anxiety, reducing their symptoms.

Of course, for a 'healthy mind in a healthy body' you need other physical contributions too – important though activity is. You need adequate sleep (see below) and a varied, balanced and healthy diet. You need to manage pain or any ongoing medical problems. All this can help you feel more confident, relaxed and in control.

We know that feeling in control, as far as possible, is important for mental well-being and 'helplessness' is a potent factor undermining it. So being informed and in control of health-related decisions (see Chapter 8) has a real part to play in mental well-being.

How does physical activity enhance mind and mood?

To be completely honest we don't know precisely. We know there is an *association* between cardiovascular exercise and improved cognitive function and mood, but how it works is still not fully understood. Better blood circulation to the brain is likely to be part of the explanation. And there are some interesting possibilities for how physical activity might boost mood.

Your body chemistry

Your body produces many different chemicals that affect mood, including endorphins, serotonins and adrenaline. Endorphins are mood enhancing and can help with pain too.

Serotonins are some of the substances our brain cells make to communicate with each other. Exercise may increase the serotonin available to your brain tissue. Concentrating the brain's own serotonin levels is the way some anti-depressants work.

Adrenaline is a hormone that stimulates your heart and circulation, makes you more alert and boosts your mental activity. In fact, adrenaline is your 'fight and flight' chemical: evolved to help your rapid escape from dangerous situations.

Simple ways

Keeping physically active is beneficial for your health, giving you strength and stamina for the rest of life. It's a much more constructive alternative to smoking or excessive drinking, if those are your current harms.

Keeping curious: learning and loving it

The connections between your brain cells are very active if you are. The brain is sometimes referred to as plastic, because of its capacity to grow ever more nerve cell branches, making new connections between cells as you use your mind and body and learn new skills. Your brain is your ultimate flexible friend, but it needs feeding, exercising and stretching every day.

What you believe about what you can do matters

Professor Patrick Rabbit reviewed the thinking skills of older people in his very readable book *The Aging Mind: An Owner's Manual*. It turns out that how we feel and what we believe about our ability DOES have an effect on our performance. If we *think* we'll succeed in something that we are capable of, then we are more likely to do just that.

If you are depressed or doing yourself down it can have a profound effect on how well you perform. If you keep saying to yourself that your mental processes aren't good enough, you will come to believe it, undermining your ability unnecessarily. You may be a bit slower than you used to be, but don't jump to conclusions about early dementia, or build false assumptions about your capability. It's much more likely that you're feeling a bit down, have lost confidence or are a bit depressed.

But if you are really worried that your thinking skills are slowing down or not working well, whatever the cause might be, see your doctor.

Feed, exercise and stretch your mind

The phrase 'use it or lose it' doesn't just apply to muscles.

Feeding your mind prevents boredom. Whether it's a good book, an art gallery, the internet or your local museum, you can stimulate and expand your mind. Hiking through interesting countryside, mindfully observing its natural history, will exercise your body, focus your mind *and* feed it. If you are continuing in the same career, consider attending courses to enrich you and prevent burn-out.

Exercising your mind regularly helps maintains it. If you don't have anything to think about, your memory and thinking become sluggish. Simple number and word games and even your daily planning and decision-making all help. You can counteract minor memory problems with lists, or tag items with funny words to fix them in your mind. Bread and milk on your mental shopping list might become 'bread bricks and mighty milk'.

Stretching your mind in new directions keeps it adaptive and forges new brain cell connections. It needs more challenging mental activity than simple rehearsal and repetition. If you find the quick crossword too easy, push those synapses and try the cryptic one instead. Playing bridge, cracking the daily sudoku in your newspaper, or learning a new language are all likely to stretch your mind and build the connections that enhance your mental ability.

Your hobby, your lifeline

Hobbies are a wonderful way of stretching, exercising and feeding your mind. They often stimulate your physical and social self too – going on a local archaeological dig, for example, will involve meeting lots of new people, and lots of bending down.

If you can't decide what to do, think about what you used to enjoy: as far back as school if necessary. Now that you might have a bit more time, why not start cooking or birdwatching again, rediscover a musical instrument – or pick up a language you started. The key thing is that it's your choice, your challenge and at your pace. You can work at it, play with it, develop it and become an expert if you want.

If you are a carer and a hobby is a distant dream – make that dream a top priority.

Maybe your first choice won't last long. That's OK – it's a stepping-stone to find what you really want to do. But find something, and build your interest. Your hobby can stretch your mind, strengthen your muscles and be an avenue to meet others if you want. In fact, **your hobby can be your lifeline,** when others seem temporarily closed off: keep yours going, or start one up if you possibly can.

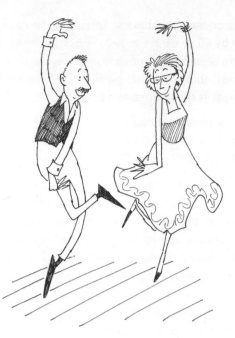

Mixing and matching your mind with others

Connecting with others helps your mind. Exchanging and debating ideas with friends is a good mental exercise. Arrange to meet an old friend for a coffee, phone someone you've been meaning to catch up with for a while, or suggest meeting up with someone you know at work or through a hobby (or exercise class).

Busting stress

Mindfulness

Simply put, mindfulness is both an attitude and a mental exercise to focus our attention on the moment we are in. The practice is often linked to a talking therapy called Cognitive Behavioural Therapy, or CBT for short. It has been very effective in helping people manage their mind and mood when things go pear-shaped with stress, anxiety, depression and other mental health problems.

Mindfulness as a technique originated in meditation within the Buddhist tradition, but it can be used whatever your framework of belief or none. A good book to look at is *Mindfulness*, by Mark Williams who, along with others, has developed the practice and application of mindfulness in the UK.

Mindfulness doesn't just belong to mental health therapy and can be used every day by all of us. It can help you experience the present moment fully, rather than steaming through the day without thought, or endlessly fretting about past things or what has not yet happened.

So mindfulness is these three things, at least:

- **Being** in the present moment.
- **Focusing** on something in the present and letting other things be.
- **Acknowledging** the moment as it is, non-judgementally.

Mindfulness can help you tap into the joy and wonder of the present. It can be practised anywhere: in a noisy station or while you walk or run. You can focus on an object in the outside world and practise letting all the other thoughts swirling in your head do what they will. You can learn to let them come or go as you repeatedly and gently bring your attention back to the object of your focus. Other things will find their own level – you can let them be for the time being.

Mindful breathing (Pearl No. 6) is a good way to start the day, and can be adapted to other situations with other objects of focus.

PEARL NO. 6: MINDFUL BREATHING

This exercise gets you to focus attentively on your breathing. It takes about 5 minutes:

✓ Place your hands on your tummy. Feel your hands move out as you breathe in and sink back as you breathe out. Focus your attention on your breathing.

✓ There may be various thoughts in your mind. Don't dwell on them – you cannot 'empty your mind'. Your thoughts and feelings will find their own level without your attention.

✓ If your attention wanders from your breathing, bring it back straight away.

✓ Continue to breathe gently and slowly, with your hands on your tummy for about 3 minutes. Keep focused on your breathing all the time.

✓ When you are ready to stop acknowledge this, and remain quiet for a further minute or two, if you can.

Mindfulness and other approaches

Mindfulness can be used alongside other therapies to help develop a calm, focused attitude of mind.

Mindfulness helps in two ways. It can help you turn away from a problem, and it can help you to turn towards it and face it. Both attitudes of mind are needed to get on with life and to solve your problem. When mindfulness helps you focus on something other than the problem itself, it allows the thoughts and feelings attached to it to rest. It enables you to turn your attention to something else.

When you turn your attention towards your problem you can begin to face it even if it makes you afraid. This helps the ferocity of anxiety and panic to ebb away. You can then manage the problem more effectively, without being overwhelmed by your emotions.

If anxiety and depression have got a grip on your mind and mood, practising mindfulness is beneficial. It complements talking therapies, particularly CBT, and reduces the risk of recurrent low mood. It's wise to see your GP to exclude things that may be making your mood worse.

One of the dangers of depression is that you withdraw into your shell, feeling as if you have no energy to do anything. It is essential to keep going with activities that help counteract the vicious cycle of low mood. Keep up your social contacts too, keep physically active, have a balanced diet and watch your alcohol intake. Consider an alcohol-free few weeks.

The following can help too:

- **Good night thoughts**: just before you go to sleep, focus on a positive thing that's happened in your day.
- **Skip it**: pick up a skipping rope – get active on the spot. And get walking.
- **The Long Goodbye**: a slow breathing technique to gently blow panic away (see Pearl 10 page 171).
- **Deep Relaxation**: deep, toe to top, relaxation (see Pearl 11 page 187).
- **The negative thought viruses**: spot them and swat them, like flies, before they undermine your self-esteem.
- **Unwanted thoughts: distance them in your mind**. Mindfully picture unwanted thoughts, and put them at an imaginary distance. Picture a window far away, and put the thoughts outside it – they can stay there.
- **Serotonin-boosting foods**: turkey, chicken, milk, eggs and nuts contain a natural substance (an essential amino acid) called tryptophan which makes serotonin and can maintain your mood. Skipping meals can affect your mood – so don't do it.

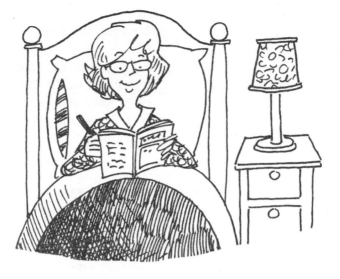

PEARL NO. 7: POSITIVE REFLECTIONS AT BEDTIME

What we think about before we go to sleep is better consolidated and better retained. So why not help positive thoughts stay in your memory - they're better than negative ones! You will need your notebook or diary, (avoid your smartphone or computer screen before sleep).

✓ Think back over the day.

✓ Pick out one or two things that you have enjoyed: however small.

✓ Write it down. And reflect on it for a minute, to appreciate the recollection.

✓ Then look ahead to tomorrow. CHOOSE ONE SMALL THING that you would *like* to do, enjoy doing and are ABLE to do, come what may. The key is to choose something achievable: like pruning a particular rose or phoning a friend you haven't spoken to for a while.

✓ Write this down and put it somewhere easy to see **first thing in the morning**.

✓ In the morning, before you look at whatever personal 'to do' list you have, have a quick look at your chosen small enjoyment for the day.

✓ Again, at the end of the day, look backwards and forwards again. Reflect on whether you did that 'nice thing' and if so, did it feel good?

If you didn't manage to do it, don't worry. Ask yourself what else happened which you enjoyed, and what the reason was for not doing what you had planned: was it unrealistic? Next day, see if you can choose something you will be able to do.

Feeling comfortable in your skin. It is exhausting and demoralising if you constantly feel distressed by the appearance of your body – but it's not uncommon. It may be simple, age-related changes that distress you, or profound changes due to surgical treatment or an accident. These adjustments can be very difficult and you may already have had counselling.

A range of approaches can help – including simply 'getting on with life' and engaging with the activities that matter to you and the social connections that can strengthen and support. Mindfulness can help you find your feet again too. You could return to your mindful mirror (see page 21) to help you regain the trust and compassion you need to find within. Instead of asking yourself questions about weight, ask yourself about your body. Choose the questions – they may be something like:

- How has my body changed?
- Is my body stopping me getting on with my life?
- Do I need help?

If you simply cannot look at yourself or engage in reflective thought about your body, it's a good indicator that you do need help to sort things out.

Living with pain is wretched, and often goes hand in hand with depression if it's unremitting. The first thing to say is that pain always needs an explanation – even if it's only 'unexplained pain' after identifiable causes have been excluded. It will be no less of a pain, but hopefully less of a worry. Do see your doctor if you have no explanation. How does mindfulness fit in? It gives you something to plant in your consciousness other than your pain. Practise mindful breathing daily, using an object you find beautiful or interesting to focus on. Let your pain sit at the back of your mind while you bring your attention to focus on the image or object you have chosen. If there are regular places you visit, plan two minutes of mindfulness there, focusing on something other than your pain.

Other good things

Get things off your chest or out of your hair

If you want to focus attentively on something but don't want to lose the thoughts that are flying around, just jot them down quickly so you can forget about them for a while, and then resume your mindfulness exercise. It's worth carrying a notebook and pencil, wherever you are.

Listen to your mood music

Music can move our mood – even against our will. Music has always had great power: to soothe, calm and comfort us.

There is something special about making your own music. It doesn't matter if you never learnt an instrument, you have your own – your voice. Give it all you've got, and SING. Sing in the shower, cooking a meal, on your way to snooker or as you walk to work. Even better, sing with others – join a choir and make music together.

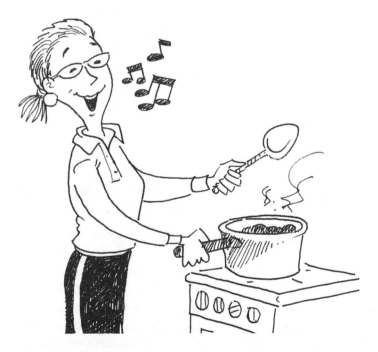

Try treats: Indulge in the pleasure principle

It's not wrong to like pleasurable things. It's part of being human. When things bring pleasure it helps us learn and relax.

Treats – simple pleasures – are simple delights; so don't forget them. They don't have to be expensive and are often better when they're not. They can be shared – a double treat and a good deed, all in one. Pick some garden flowers for the kitchen table, and some for your neighbour.

Chill out

Most of us need brief intervals to relax or let our hair down (if we still have some).

Tiny, unplanned breathing spaces to let off steam, let your hair down or just chill out for a bit, work best when there are no 'oughts' or 'shoulds' attached. If you're juggling lots of balls in the air or busy being a carer, they are rare but precious moments. Catch them when you can. A relaxing bath can be a good moment to listen to a bit of music, and make the most of that quiet 20-minute retreat. However brief, we all need them. They don't need to be costly, far away or complicated. The important thing is not to keep putting them off.

Yoga, deep relaxation (see Pearl No. 11, Chapter 7), massage and aromatherapy may all help you feel like you've had a mini holiday, especially if life is hectic.

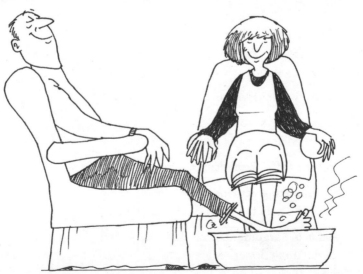

Keeping sleep sound

It is important to have adequate, regular sleep. If you are deprived of it, your mental well-being can plummet.

SLEEP HYGIENE

Here are seven things you can do to help a healthy sleeping pattern:

1. Make sure you have **regular 'getting up' times**: whatever the night was like. Don't lie in at the weekends if you can help it, it disrupts your rhythm and makes it harder to get to sleep that night.

2. Take **exercise**: get enough during the day and you'll feel ready for bed by the end of it.

3. Have some **'wind-down'** time; relax during the last hour before bedtime.

4. Make sure you have a **cool but not cold bedroom** – about 18°C (65°F) helps sleep.

5. Make sure you have a **dark, quiet bedroom** – wear eye shades or ear plugs.

6. **Avoid sleep disturbance**: don't use your computer screen, TV, or back-lit mobile phone late at night. Drift off to sleep with a good book instead.

7. Finding your **healthy weight** improves your sleep quality. Excess weight, especially obesity, causes snoring, and sleep apnoea (interruption of your breathing during sleep), which reduces sleep quality.

And here are six things to avoid:

1. **Don't have long daytime naps**: naps lasting more than about 45 minutes disrupt your sleep cycle.

2. **Don't drink caffeine or alcohol late at night**.

3. **Over-stimulating activities** late in the evening – like watching a thriller film – gets the brain in 'active' mode.

4. **Try and avoid arguments** with family and friends (sometimes easier said than done). 'Make up' if you can. If not, flag and resolve in the morning.

5. **Avoid lots of fluid after 7pm**: it makes you get up during the night.

6. **Try not to take sleeping tablets** – unless you have a severe, short-term need. They cause daytime drowsiness and are often addictive.

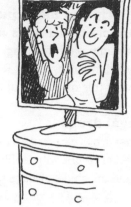

If you really can't get to sleep ...

... deal with it as simply as you can. If you're still awake after about 30 minutes of trying to nod off, get up quietly. Jot down racing thoughts in a notebook or diary (not an electronic device) and put them away until the next waking day.

When awake, think of the time as a temporary 'wind-down' phase. Don't watch TV or DVDs – read a book or listen to quiet music through headphones so you don't disturb anyone. Don't try to sort the problems you didn't sort out yesterday. Don't check your e-mails. After about 30–45 minutes go through your regular bedtime routine again: brushing your teeth, for example. It's very behavioural and often works well after a few tries.

If worrying about problems is stopping you sleep, plan to sort these out as soon as possible.

Stay out of harm's way

Dependencies and addictions

Destructive habits and dependencies still cause harm in our 60s. Alcohol excess is common in us baby boomers. Keep your intake within safe limits to avoid serious consequences (see Chapter 5 on you and your liver).

Fewer of us smoke, but if you do – it's time to stop. See page 106 for some advice.

Prescription medicines

Drugs prescribed to us for pain relief, anxiety and sleep problems are commonly habit-forming, and long after the original need has passed we may still be using them. Review your medication regularly with your GP to prevent this or sort it out (see Chapter 8).

Illegal drugs

Illegal drugs can cause a lot of harm, even if some give short-term pleasure. Whether or not you dabbled with them in your hippy years, have used them on and off since, or have taken them up more recently, they can harm your health in a variety of ways.

If, despite the obvious dangers and your best intentions, you are still taking illegal drugs of any kind, you should STOP NOW. Here are four good helplines to try:

- Your GP surgery.
- Narcotics Anonymous (www.na.org).
- NHS Choices (www.nhs.uk) – see the pages on help for illegal drug use.
- FRANK (www.talktofrank.com) – a national drug education service.

Non substance-based addictions

Whatever the addictive behaviour is, it has a kick and a thrill for the person doing it, which is reinforced the more you do it. If it starts to take over your life and prevent you from doing other things it is becoming a problem. The commonest non substance-based addictive behaviour is gambling. It is more common and much easier with the internet.

If you or others are worried that you might have a gambling problem it is worth doing something about it. It is possible to break the habit and taking the first step to get help is often half the battle.

Look at the NHS Choices site (www.nhs.uk). You can refer yourself to the NHS National Problem Gambling Clinic (020-7381-772). You need a referral form, which you can get online at gambling.cnwl@nhs.net. There are other sources of help too: Gam Care (0808-8020-133, www. gamcare.org.uk), and Gamblers Anonymous (www.gamblersanonymous. org.uk).

RESOLUTIONS

Here are some resolutions to consider for every day:

✓ I will try to meet with someone I know or am getting to know.

✓ I will do some physical activity that makes me a bit breathless.

✓ I will try to learn or develop something new.

✓ I will try to do at least one good deed for someone else.

✓ I will focus mindfully for 5 minutes on something in the 'present'.

KEEPING YOUR METABOLISM HEALTHY

By the time we have reached our 60s, a lot of us have been inactive for too long and consuming more food than necessary. The result? More than two thirds of us are overweight or obese: and it piles up and up. This has serious consequences for our health, including type 2 diabetes and raised levels of unhelpful cholesterol, which increases the risk of heart attacks and other problems. Being overweight increases your blood pressure and raises the risk of a stroke. So we need to understand what happens.

Fat facts

Being overweight can lead to something called the 'metabolic syndrome', which is worth knowing about so you can prevent it or roll it back as much as you can if you have it. The fat that builds up inside and around our tummies is particularly bad news for our health. It can lead to type 2 diabetes which can affect the heart, eyes, kidneys and nerves, as well as lots of other problems that might occur even before diabetes has developed. So be a trendsetter, roll back your tummy fat.

Fat is the storehouse for all the extra calories that you haven't burnt up. We store the extra calories we consume as fat under our skin, inside our tummy, in and around our organs, and around our middle. If we don't burn up our calories by keeping our bodies on the go and keeping active, they just get converted to fat that builds up and up over the years (see the box on biscuits on page 79).

We need a little layer of fat under our skin for insulation and protection. We don't want our bones poking out and getting knocked and bumped every time we move. But beyond this, fat starts to build up unhelpfully, and when it builds up in and around our middle, causing what we used to call rather affectionately our 'middle-aged spread', it causes the apple body shape that signals excess weight and obesity. Tummy fat is bad for your health, so let's look at why.

Fat certainly doesn't sit there doing nothing, which is what we used to think. Being overweight or obese does all this:

- **It increases the load on your joints**: bad for joint pain and arthritis.
- **It slows you down**, as your heart has to work harder to keep you moving.
- **It makes you walk differently**, stressing your joints in other ways.
- **It increases the risk of many cancers**. Cancer Research UK (www.cancerresearchuk.org) reports that obesity is a major preventable cause of many cancers, and increases the risk of each of the following: breast (after the menopause), bowel, womb, gullet, stomach, pancreatic, kidney and liver cancer.

As tummy fat starts to build up, it can lead to:

- Rising blood sugar levels and eventually type 2 diabetes.
- Increased levels of unhelpful cholesterol (the LDL type, see Chapter 5 on your heart) that clogs up arteries and cause heart attacks and strokes.

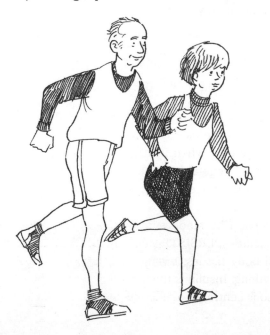

In other words, your increasing tummy fat works against you. How bad is that? Let's look more closely.

Because smoking levels have decreased overall in the population, especially in our age group, obesity has now overtaken smoking as the leading causes of ill heath in the population as a whole. It remains true that if you do smoke, quitting smoking is still likely to be the single most important thing you could do to benefit your health.

However, sugary drinks, and sugar and fat-rich foods (biscuits, cakes, pies and pastries, sweets, chocolates, processed and fatty meats) load us with extra calories we don't use up, contributing to excess weight and obesity – which works against you as it accumulates. Alcohol is a major source of surplus calories too, and brings all the other problems that occur when it's consumed in excess. Even on its own, but usually hand in hand with the rich foods listed above, alcohol contributes to an expanding belly.

Beer bellies are more likely to lead to lower levels of testosterone too – not good news for libido (see Chapter 5).

To understand the 'metabolic syndrome' and how to reverse it by losing weight, we'll need to mention a few things you will have heard of (like insulin, blood sugar, cholesterol, metabolism and metabolic rate) but, unless you have diabetes already, you may not be absolutely clear why they're important or why they are relevant now.

Metabolic health

Glucose

The body needs glucose as its 'moment by moment' energy source. The brain uses glucose as its energy supply, as does all your body. But your body works best when it makes its own glucose, out of a healthy diet: wholegrain, vegetables and fruits. When it can do this (on a Mediterranean diet, for example), it's easy for the body to keep blood sugar at safe levels.

Blood glucose (the blood sugar we're talking about) HAS to stay at safe levels, because PERSISTENT HIGH BLOOD GLUCOSE (diabetes) is TOXIC to all body tissues: brain, heart, arteries, kidneys, eyes, muscles, nerves, everything. Insulin is the hormone keeping blood sugar levels safe and steady, so is central to metabolic health.

Cholesterol

Your body needs cholesterol. It is a type of body fat (or LIPID), found in every single cell in your body. It's needed for many important body chemicals. But, like glucose, the body needs to keep safe levels of circulating cholesterol, otherwise things go wrong (like arteries getting clogged). It does this most easily when it makes its own cholesterol from healthy sources, like oily fish (no more than a couple of portions a week), plant oils like olive oil, nuts, seeds and eggs.

Cholesterol is transported in the blood in two forms: High Density Lipoprotein (HDL) and Low Density Lipoprotein (LDL). The HDL acts to protect the heart and blood vessels; the LDL works with other body chemicals to clog up the linings of arteries and make them inflamed – so is bad. When the body has **lots** of saturated and trans fats **all the time** (animal fats like lard, rich dairy full creams, butter and hard cheeses, and industrially hardened trans fats), all of which are found in biscuits, cakes, pastries and most processed meals, more LDL cholesterol circulates (very bad news). But when it has the healthy plant and oily fish sources mentioned, it makes more of the circulation-friendly HDL cholesterol.

Insulin

This is your body's chief blood sugar regulator, and is made in your pancreas. It helps regulate levels of blood cholesterol too. The body depends on insulin to keep blood glucose (and blood fats) at safe levels.

Safe and steady blood sugar levels

If you eat too much food – more than you burn up – all the time, then the metabolic system and insulin from the pancreas, have to work double – if not triple – time to keep pace and store it away outside the circulation, converting all the excess calories into stored body fat. The body's blood glucose MUST be kept at safe, steady levels, to stop it rising persistently, harming the circulation and all the vital organs.

Insulin resistance

This is at the heart of the so-called 'metabolic syndrome'. For reasons we still don't understand, when most people get more and more overweight and gather more and more stored central body fat, the metabolic system (liver, muscles and fat) becomes resistant to insulin. Once the metabolism is less sensitive to the regulatory role of insulin, blood glucose levels and blood fat levels rise – causing a spiral of more insulin release to compensate for its dwindling effects. This is what leads to heart attacks, strokes, type 2 diabetes and all its complications.

A body fit for purpose

Metabolic health means a body fit for purpose: active, energetic and free from excess weight. Your metabolism is the chemistry that keeps you alive and your metabolic system ensures sufficient energy (battery power) for this and all you do.

And because what goes in doesn't come out, what goes in is *either* **USED** *or* **STORED**. The human tank expands to take all you put in it. So there is no alternative. There are only three possibilities at the end of each day:

- **Energy balance** – a 'good metabolic system' – eating what your body needs, but not too much, or too little.
- **Excess supply** – you eat more than you need – so you store the excess as fat.
- **Excess demand** – you eat less than your body needs, forcing it to use up some of your fat supplies – fine in moderation if you're trying to lose weight.

And it's all about energy so it can ALL be measured in the same units – calories.

These are your metabolic organs:

- **Your liver**: your processor, sending glucose and other nutrients, to your body.
- **Your skeletal muscle**: great at using energy.
- **Your fat (adipose) tissue**: think of this as a thin layer of thermal underwear when you're healthy.

The two main things driving your metabolic rate are the amount of activity you do and the hormones from your endocrine system The most important hormone controlling your metabolic rate is thyroxine, from your thyroid gland, which increases your rate of using up stored energy. Its level is balanced automatically by the brain (unless something goes wrong with your thyroid gland).

Other factors, such as your age and sex hormones, have a small effect too.

As you get older, your metabolic rate drops fractionally year by year. Your sex hormones normally increase your metabolic rate slightly – mainly by building up your muscles, which are key to burning up energy. As levels of sex hormone drop slightly in men with age, and more significantly in women after the menopause, metabolic rate drops a little as well. This means that you **have** to exercise more, or consume a little less, or both, year by year, to keep to your healthy weight.

Your lowest rate of energy use (your basal metabolic rate) is when you're sleeping. The rate gets a little higher when you're awake but resting (your resting metabolic rate), and gets higher and higher the more activity you consciously do (your active, or total metabolic rate). So you can see just how important your lifestyle is to your metabolism.

There is no perfect way of measuring whether you are overweight, but your body mass index is one way. With few exceptions, the higher your BMI, the more overweight you are. Another simple guide is to look mindfully in your mirror, as you did at the end of Chapter 1 (see page 21). It's not precise, but it tells you a lot of what you need to know.

YOUR BMI

Your BMI is the ratio of your weight to the square of your height. These are the ranges used by the NHS, and www.nhs.uk has excellent pages on BMI, with a calculator that works with imperial or metric measures:

Category	BMI Guide Range (NHS)
Underweight	Less than 18.5
Normal	18.5–24.9*
Overweight	25–29.9
Obese	30 and more

*If you are Asian or black, your healthy BMI will be nearer to 23, to offset a higher genetic risk of metabolic syndrome (see page 80).

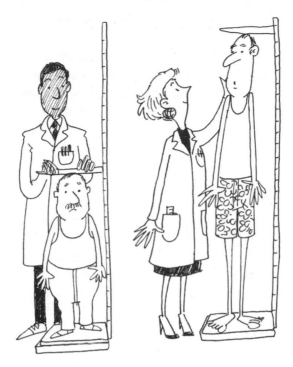

Too much weight, raised blood glucose and raised LDL cholesterol is your metabolic system under stress. Metabolic Syndrome often comes hand in hand with high blood pressure. Chronic stress – whether physical (as in this central example of expanding fat) mental or mechanical – always causes harm. And this is why you need to bust the stress of metabolic ill health by losing your excess weight and finding your healthy weight. The box below shows how even a few excess calories each day can mount up month by month and year by year, building excess weight and obesity almost without you noticing.

DOWN WITH COLA AND BISCUITS; UP WITH EXERCISE

Just over one chocolate digestive (or 6 level teaspoons of sugar or 100 kilocalories) excess to your needs each day, over the course of a year, is equivalent to about 4 kilograms of fat. That's just over half a stone. The calories-to-fat conversion is only a rough guide, but it's good enough.

If this happens over 10 years, during your 50s for example – it can mount up to approximately 40kg of excess fat (that's just over 6 stone). So if you were a 50-year-old woman weighing 9 stone ten years ago, but you consumed 100 calories excess to your need every day for a decade, you would arrive at 60 weighing about 15 stone with a BMI of 37 – significantly obese.

If you're not a biscuit eater, think of a 330ml can of cola – 140 kilocalories. It wouldn't take as long as 10 years to get to 15 stone if you drink a can of cola excess to your needs each day. And this is exactly what happens to many of us. And if it's happened to you, *you* can reverse it, by burning up your stores and avoiding sugary drinks to lose weight. Down with cola; up with exercise.

And as we mentioned at the start of the chapter, being overweight contributes to high blood pressure, especially when excess calories come from alcohol (which pushes up blood pressure additionally while in the body). And as we have also seen, not only is the 'metabolic syndrome' a physically stressed state, it links in with other stresses too.

A major hidden factor in this unhelpful cycle of metabolic stress is often mental stress, where loss of self-esteem and depression drive over-eating, as well as over-drinking, smoking and inactivity. When you get right down to it, mental stress may even be the root cause of metabolic stress in some people. The reason excess weight leads to metabolic stress in 'most of us' and not 'everyone' is down to genetics.

Most of us are genetically at risk of insulin resistance and a stressed metabolism if we gain weight. But a lucky few have a genetic make-up that protects them from the metabolic stress of being overweight. But at the other end of the spectrum, a very unlucky few get metabolically stressed even at a normal healthy weight. For these people, medication at an early stage is essential to protect them from their increased risk of type 2 diabetes and heart disease, or help them if have it already.

Different beasts

It's important to distinguish between type 2 diabetes, which usually develops in adults and is predominantly lifestyle related, from type 1 diabetes, which usually develops in children and adolescents, and has nothing to do with lifestyle.

But once diabetes has arrived, both types risk complications leading to heart attacks, stroke, kidney, eye and nerve damage, and need treatment to avoid further complications. People with type 1 diabetes always needs insulin. Those with type 2 diabetes may end up needing it if their underlying lifestyle and excess weight are not reversed, because the pancreas cannot keep up with the increasing demand for insulin.

Once you've found your healthy weight, or if you're there already, the best thing is to stick to a Mediterranean diet (see below) with plenty of vegetables, fruit and fibre.

Finding your healthy weight

Just 4 kilograms weight loss makes a big difference to your risk of type 2 diabetes – one piece of research showed that it can reduce your 'relative' risk by 58 per cent. Problems such as obesity and type 2 diabetes are both common and serious, so a relative risk reduction on this scale is very important indeed. Remember, every bit of exercise helps and every bit of weight loss helps. When you've found your healthy weight – keep it. Keep your energy supply and demand balanced, keep active and only consume what you burn up.

It's not about a 'diet'– it's about eating healthily. Healthy eating is about healthy quantity as well as nutrition. Lose weight steadily as part of a healthy plan (not a crash course, which can end up in a nasty cycle of dieting, failing and depression). Here are some good tips for losing weight the healthy way (see also Pearl No. 8: Mindful Eating, on page 86):

LOSE WEIGHT THE HEALTHY WAY

✓ **Eat regularly:** don't skip breakfast, you'll snack all morning if you do.

✓ **Eat healthily:** less is more when you need to lose weight.

✓ **Keep the balance right:** even when you reduce the overall quantities.

✓ **Keep up your fibre:** it fills you up (eat more porridge, wholegrains, vegetables, fruit, nuts, seeds).

✓ **Eat lots of vegetables and fruit:** five portions a day, but not fruit juices (too sugary) and avoid the added sugars of sweets, chocolates, biscuits and cakes and cereal bars.

✓ **Chew well and slowly:** and put your cutlery down between mouthfuls.

✓ **Drink sufficient water or unsweetened watery drinks:** cut out ALL sweetened drinks and count your alcohol calories.

✓ **Stop eating** before you're absolutely full (see mindful eating on page 86)

The next steps

If you are significantly overweight, try losing 4 kilograms over two months. Your gradual weight loss will lower your risk of type 2 diabetes (or reduce its impact) and you will be encouraged to decide on the next steps in two months' time.

Weight loss clinics and clubs

These work well for many people. The combination of social support, specific guidance and calorie counting can help. The caution is that they can emphasise a prescribed 'diet' and sometimes also special 'diet' products. This doesn't always integrate so well with long-term healthy eating. But you know what works well for you.

Get active: use your muscles!

Remember that small bursts of exercise all add up. You need to burn off the calorie store that you've built up over the years. So get active and get walking. You need cardiovascular, stamina-boosting exercise AND strengthening exercises, mixing them up in a combination that suits you. Brisk walking, especially when mixed with a few bursts of power-producing exercise, like raising weights or a series of ten star jumps, will help you burn up excess fat not just when you're active but when you're resting too (by raising your basal and resting metabolic rate, see page 78).

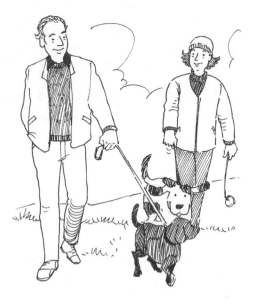

Remember your Attitude?

Be compassionate with yourself. Remember your mindful mirror? If you are overweight you need a gentle, non-judgemental attitude towards it. Fixating negatively on your weight wastes valuable emotional energy. Think of eating healthily and losing excess weight as a job to do, not a stick to beat yourself with. Remember, your weight is your weight, not your worth.

And encourage yourself

Every bit of excess weight lost helps. Your body is already working to undo damage to your metabolic system from excess body fat. It's a win–win situation. If you have the 'metabolic syndrome' or type 2 diabetes and are on medication – please don't stop it. But if you increase your activity, lose your excess weight and keep it off, you may not need medication. That is real and realistic. Aim high. You can do it!

What is a healthy diet?

Although it is often easier said than done, a healthy diet is one in which you eat what you need, and no more. But, by following the advice here you will be able to come up with an appropriate and tasty diet that will help you find your healthy weight and maintain it without dieting and without too much trouble.

Your energy supply should come mainly (about two thirds) from wholegrain carbohydrates. The remaining third comes from protein and fats, ideally more protein than fat. The exact amount you need to keep your healthy weight will vary from person to person, depending on your healthy BMI. The quantity and balance will vary from day to day, but over the course of a week your average daily energy consumption should match your energy output.

Eat real food – Mediterranean style

You need (at least) five portions of vegetables and fruit each day: orange, red, yellow, green and blue, deep dark violet, all the colours of the rainbow. Think peppers, carrots, red cabbage, tomatoes, broccoli, rocket, spinach, butternut squash, beetroot, and so on – the more colourful the better. Steamed, grated into a salad, flash fried in a stir-fry or roasted in a drizzle of olive oil.

And fish: white, and oily (two portions a week), or a vegetarian alternative like soya and walnuts to provide essential protein and omega fats.

A little fat helps you feel satisfied, but it's calorie rich, however it comes. So use the minimum necessary for cooking and drizzling on salads, and always go for olive oil rather than saturated fats where you can. Go for balance, use skimmed or semi-skimmed milk and cottage cheese, with very small amounts of the harder cheeses for taste and variety – a bit of what you like for flavour is fine.

(The information given here is STILL the advice from the British Heart Foundation [www.bhf.org.uk] despite the recent media flurry. See Which is worse, fat or sugar? on page 85.)

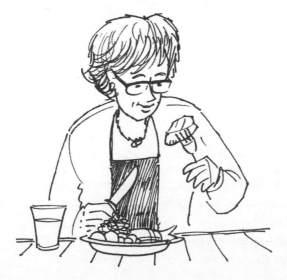

MORE AND LESS FOR A HEALTHY METABOLISM

Eat and drink more ...	Eat and drink less ...
• **vegetables and fruit** (go for the brightly coloured ones).	• **biscuits, cakes, sweet milk chocolate and sweets.**
• **water** – about 6–8 tall glasses or mugs daily: more if it's hot weather and you've done sweaty exercise.	• **sugary drinks and fruit juice** • **alcohol** – 21 units per week for a man, 14 for a woman.
• **fibre** – wholegrain, nuts and seeds.	• **refined foods, white rice and bread.**
• **balance** – enough, but not too much, protein and essential fat: soy, lentils, nuts, semi-skimmed milk, white fish, eggs, and oily fish twice a week.	• **red meat and preserved meats:** sausages, hams and salamis.
• **variety** in your diet to get vitamins calcium, iron, and minerals into your diet.	• **less** monotony • **less** strict dieting.

Which is worse, fat or sugar?

Added sugars and high fat foods are both unhelpful, for several reasons. They are calorie and energy rich, so quickly add up to more than we need and more than we burn up, leading to excess calories and weight. Olive oil is just as calorific as saturated fat but saturated fats push up the LDL levels and so are much more harmful to the heart and circulation than olive oil and other unsaturated oils (like sunflower, corn, almond, rapeseed and peanut oil). Of course, if it's in excess of your energy needs, olive oil, like any other source of calories, will be converted to fat.

The problem with sugary foods and drinks, apart from clocking up more unnecessary calories, is that it leads to a big glucose load released quickly into your circulation after digestion. This stimulates your pancreas to produce a much higher burst of insulin than would be needed with a smaller load.

But if you get more and more overweight, your metabolic system becomes less and less sensitive to insulin, so needs more and more of it. The poor pancreas cannot keep pace, and so begins the vicious cycle.

Sugar is absolutely everywhere. In real terms, it's the thing that we are all most exposed to, however hard we try to avoid it. There are alarming amounts of sugar in sugary drinks. It's in almost all processed and low-fat foods, and most added sugar is surplus to our needs. The problem is that sugar is addictive and it's hard to say no. It's not surprising we've started to say that sugar is the real problem, and not fat.

So you absolutely don't need to add sugar to your diet! The occasional bit of sugar in a celebration cake is fine, but keep it special. A healthy diet needs pure, clear water rather than sugary drinks or alcohol.

PEARL NO. 8: MINDFUL EATING

Being mindful when you eat can help you lose weight. Remember that you should aim for a varied, balanced diet to provide your body with the essential nutrients it needs. Here are some suggestions to help you enjoy your mindful meal and lose weight:

✓ Make sure all you need is on the table. Sit where it is bright if you can.

✓ To avoid second helpings, put a small portion of your prepared food onto a spare plate, and put it to one side for tomorrow – or for a guest.

✓ Have a glass of water and avoid wine if working or driving.

✓ Look at the colour and arrangement of your food, give thanks for it.

✓ Let the aroma of your food waft towards you, enjoy it.

✓ Eat slowly and chew carefully – notice the texture and taste change.

✓ If you're full – put your fork down and push the plate away. If you're almost full – do the same.

✓ Focus quietly on the feeling of fullness. Let the sensation sink in.

Red flags

We have talked positively about your metabolic health, how to eat well, lose weight and avoid the metabolic syndrome. However, you should always be aware of the following red flags:

- **Thirst, constantly passing urine and recurrent skin infections** are potential symptoms of diabetes, so it is always wise to see your GP if you are suffering from them.

- **Gaining significant weight around your tummy** is a warning of obesity and the metabolic syndrome or the side effect of medicines: discuss it with your doctor and get cracking losing weight and getting active.
- **And if you are gaining weight, sluggish, constipated and feeling the cold**: see your GP to check your thyroid gland isn't underactive, it is vital to pick this up as early as possible.
- **Weight loss: if it's not deliberate** it is essential to see your GP. Usually it's straightforward, but an overactive thyroid, or cancer, needs ruling out.
- **Feeling tired all the time**: if persistent, this is a red flag. See the section on muscle strength in Chapter 2.

RESOLUTIONS

Here are some resolutions to consider for everyday use.

✓ I will eat a varied, balanced Mediterranean type diet.

✓ I will find my healthy weight, and keep it.

✓ I will walk as much as I can and as briskly as I can.

✓ I will not drink sugary drinks or eat sweets, or give them to my family.

✓ I will report unexplained weight loss promptly.

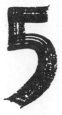

TAKE CARE OF YOUR ...
BITS

This chapter is about taking care of your body, so you can keep it in good condition to meet the challenges of life that you will encounter in your 60s. Your body deserves the very best you can give it and the advice contained here will help you provide it. However, if you think there might be a more serious problem than an age-related change, don't let it fester. Think about it 'mindfully' if you can. Talk about it with a trusted friend or family member. Try looking at useful websites like NHS Choices at www.nhs.uk, patient.co.uk, or www.healthtalk.org. But if you think there's a problem that needs discussion with a health professional then please do seek help, and talk to your pharmacist, practice nurse or GP as appropriate.

Remember the maxim: IF IN DOUBT – CHECK IT OUT!

Some of your bits need daily care: your teeth, your feet and your skin, for example. You also need to eat a varied, balanced and appropriately sized daily diet for your individual need. You will benefit from keeping as physically and mentally active as you can each day, doing 10 minutes Triple S exercises (see page 34–46), and keep connected with friends and family. Other bits need more general care. This is about how to deal with the age-related changes your bits (and you) might encounter and what you can do about them.

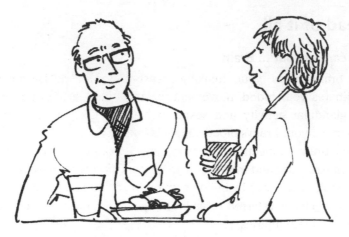

Red flags: the bleeding obvious

It may be helpful to pick out five emergencies here, in case you're a reader who skips to sections only when needed, and might miss out on useful tips upfront. Each section has its own red flag list, however, and important symptoms will soon become clear.

Five red flags that need immediate help (call 999 or 112 on your mobile):

1. **Chest pain for more than 10 minutes**: sudden and severe at rest, or not stopping if you do rest.
2. **Choking** or you can't get your breath.
3. **Stroke:** if your **F**ace droops to one side, or you lose power in an **A**rm or leg or suddenly lose your **S**peech, **T**ime is of the essence (F.A.S.T).
4. **Bleeding** from where you shouldn't, **999 if it's heavy**. (If it's not heavy, discuss the problem with your duty GP the same day, as they can direct you to the best care should you need hospital help.)
5. **A fall injuring a limb –** causing severe pain that is worse if you try to move your limb, especially if it's in your hip or leg and you cannot bear weight.

Ahead of it all

Take care of your ... Brain

Your brain helps your thinking, reasoning and decision-making. It coordinates your mood, movement, balance, bladder and bowel control, your glandular activity and sexual behaviour. Oxygen is critical to its function, so your brain's blood supply is vital.

Your brain connections are very flexible. Given the right stimulation, relevant exercises and motivation, the brain can often compensate for loss of function in one area by building up brain cell connections nearby, which take over. This is referred to as brain plasticity and helps recovery from stroke and brain injuries.

Age-related changes

Ageing leads to a slow, natural loss of brain cells (neurons) from early infancy. This contributes to slight reductions in speed of recall and mental processing. As far as we know, brain cells are not replaced when they die, so it's important to make the most of those you have and prevent further loss by every means possible. But you can grow the connections (synapses) between the millions of cells in your grey matter by increasing your physical and mental activity and having a healthy diet.

Age-related brain changes are the effects of risk factors. Your genetics, social circumstances and environment undoubtedly play a part. But lifestyle is important and contributes to preventable brain disease, mainly cerebrovascular. This can show itself suddenly, with a stroke, or slowly and progressively like vascular dementia.

Cerebrovascular disease is when the arteries supplying the brain are narrowed or blocked, reducing its blood supply. Sometimes, tiny blood clots can form in the heart, or inside big arteries, and travel to smaller arteries right inside the brain. This can cause mini, or more major strokes (see page 94). If you have clot-busting treatment in time (four and a half hours max), it can prevent long-term disability. Cerebrovascular disease can also cause lots of very tiny strokes that are hardly noticed, if not missed altogether, but contribute to vascular dementia.

Dementia is severe and progressive memory loss with movement, balance and sometimes behavioural problems. It can occur in our 60s, but is not common until our 80s and 90s. Grey matter is lost at a much greater rate than with simple ageing, and probably by a range of different mechanisms. Not all dementias, or progressive diseases like Parkinson's disease, are preventable by lifestyle.

What you can do for your brain

There are lots of things you can do to protect your brain cells and grow new connections. You can:

1. Boost your brain function and reduce your risk of stroke and dementia.

We saw in Chapter 2 that physical activity alone reduces the risk of stroke and dementia by 30 per cent each. Add to that all the following benefits, and it's a no-brainer. Your NHS health check can find out if anything more than lifestyle changes are needed, particularly if you have a family history of stroke or dementia. You may be recommended to take cholesterol-lowering medication (see page 108) if your risk is high. Aspirin (or similar drugs) may be recommended if you've had a mini or a major stroke before.

- **Clock up your cardiovascular exercise**: do your 150 minutes of moderately intense activity, it can help reduce your blood pressure too.
- **Stop smoking**: the more you try the more likely you are to stop. See lung health (page 105) and the NHS smoke-free website (www. nhs.uk/smokefree).
- **Check your blood pressure**: if it's high get help to reduce it (see page 105), with medication if necessary.
- **Report an irregular pulse** to rule out atrial fibrillation (see page 102), which causes clots that block the blood supply to your brain (causing stroke). Please see your GP to exclude this and find out whether you need stroke prevention treatment.
- **Lose excess weight:** this helps reduce your blood pressure and improves your metabolic health too (see page 75).
- **Eat bright-coloured vegetables and fruit**: keep up your five a day.

And don't forget that stretching and exercising your mind, looking after your mood, busting stress and keeping socially involved is all helpful to brain function.

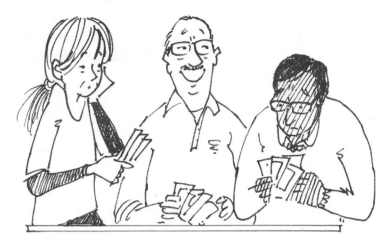

2. **Protect your brain from injury**

- **Alcohol**: is rapidly absorbed into the brain, impairing reasoning, judgement and balance – don't drink and drive. In excess it causes damage, so keep it in safe limits (see page 120). A few **prescribed drugs** may increase dementia risk *if* used in high doses for a long time. Please discuss any concerns with your GP *before* stopping prescribed medication.
- **Accidents**: ALWAYS wear your seat belt, including on coaches, and your helmet on bikes and motorbikes. If you knock your head and think you may be concussed, seek medical attention. Ask someone to check on you from time to time over the next ten days in case of delayed symptoms (vomiting, double vision, drowsiness) suggesting a blood clot pressing on the brain. This is VERY IMPORTANT IF YOU LIVE ALONE.
- **Reduce the risk of falls**. Tie your shoelaces. Practise your balance skills (see page 45) and strengthen your body core and leg muscles. Check your vision (see page 95). Check your medicines, and reduce your need for sleeping tablets – they make you wobbly at night and in the morning.
- **Carbon monoxide poisoning**. If you have gas heating and it goes wrong, carbon monoxide can build up in the air. This is dangerous if you breathe it in, as it makes it difficult for oxygen to circulate in your blood. You can't smell it, so install a carbon monoxide alarm to give you early warning.

3. **Act F.A.S.T** if you think you're having a stroke

If you or someone near you notices that one side of your face (**F**) has suddenly 'drooped' – the corner of your mouth doesn't lift when you smile, you lose power in your arm (**A**) and/or your leg, or you suddenly lose your speech (**S**) you may have had a stroke, then time (**T**) is of the essence. You need to get to hospital **F.A.S.T (within 4 and a half hours max)** for possible clot-busting treatment. Dial **999**, (or **112** on your mobile).

Red flags

- **Possible stroke**: think **F.A.S.T– dial 999** (or **112** on your mobile).
- **Sudden loss of consciousness**: you may realise you have been unconscious (or you may see that someone else is). You (or they) need urgent medical help.
- **Persistent memory problems** and near misses (like a pan burning dry on the stove) are more likely to be due to anxiety or depression. But occasionally they indicate early dementia. Please see your GP, and take someone with you if possible.
- **Difficulty with movements**: if you have unexplained difficulty getting up out of a chair, a shuffling walk, or a tremor of your hand when you're resting, it might be early Parkinson's disease. Please see your GP.
- **Risk factors for stroke**: if you know you have several risk factors and haven't discussed them with your GP – then please do it now.

RESOLUTIONS

✓ I will do my recommended 150 minutes of active physical exercise each week.

✓ I will get help to quit smoking.

✓ I will think F.A.S.T if I or someone else seems to be having a stroke.

✓ I will keep an eye on my blood pressure, and report an irregular pulse.

✓ I will keep learning, practise mindfulness, manage stress and look after my emotional well-being.

Take care of your ... Vision

Vision (and hearing) are vitally important to independence and connectedness with others, and so are central to mental well-being and keeping you active and safe.

Your vision needs your eye and brain to work together to make sense of what you see. In fact, the back of the eye, the retina, is a part of the brain and a window on its health. Your optician takes advantage of this at your eye check. It provides lots of clues to visual problems, as well as to the health of your brain circulation.

Age-related changes

The most common change, affecting nearly everyone from the age of about 40, is age-related long sightedness (or *presbyopia*). This is due to the loss of elasticity of the lens, making reading difficult because the lens resists the shape change required to focus close up.

Cataracts (clouding of the lens), and **age-related macular degeneration**, (AMD) can occur in our 60s but more commonly develop in our 70s and beyond. AMD makes distance vision, fine detail close vision and colour perception difficult, as it affects the central, most sensitive, part of the retina. It needs careful management by an eye specialist.

The commonest age-related changes in our 60s after presbyopia are those due to medical conditions:

- **Diabetes** (the most common cause of blindness in the UK).
- **High blood pressure** (if poorly controlled and very high it damages the retina causing visual loss or double vision).
- **Glaucoma**: where the pressure within the eye is raised and can, if progressive, cause visual loss.

Diabetic eye changes can happen at any age with either type of diabetes, depending how long it's been present and how difficult it has been to control. Diabetes affects the macular part of the retina, causing reduced close up as well as distance vision, and also earlier cataract formation.

What you can do for your vision

1. The most important preventive health steps are to ensure:

- **A healthy lifestyle**: stop smoking, have your five a day fresh fruit and vegetables, especially the brightly coloured ones, keep a healthy weight and keep your blood pressure controlled.

- **Using sunglasses in bright sunlight** and NEVER look directly at the sun – it damages the retina at the back of the eye, and contributes to cataracts.
- **If diabetic, keep it well controlled.** If it's type 2, try to roll it back (see page 216).

2. For early detection of problems make sure you have:

- **Regular eye checks** to update your spectacles prescription and check the pressure in your eyes to rule out glaucoma. If you have a family history, this will be done annually. An optician will also check your retina for evidence of medical conditions, like high blood pressure, diabetes, raised cholesterol and other problems.
- **An annual retinal screening**, if you are diabetic. This is important as it can pick up any early treatment that might be needed.

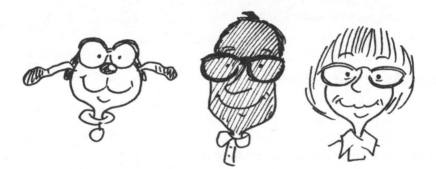

If glaucoma or a cataract is diagnosed, it does not mean you automatically have to have treatment. Discuss the issues carefully with your optician and GP.

Red flags

- **Gradual loss of vision**: get your eyes tested (you need to be able to read a car number plate at 20.5 metres (just over 21 yards). Usually spectacles need changing, but occasionally more serious causes need specialist assessment.
- **Sudden loss of vision**: partial or complete, with or without flashing lights, requires emergency attendance at a specialist eye hospital, or general A&E.
- **Persistent flashing lights**, usually after a large shower of 'floaters' like a waterfall in your vision (indicating bleeding into the jelly

material of the eye) is another same-day emergency. It may be the development of a small retinal tear.

- **Sudden or recent onset of double vision**, particularly with a severe headache in your temples. This may flag inflammation of the arteries supplying your retina (or other serious problems) and it's ESSENTIAL to see your GP the same day. If you can't, go directly to A&E.

RESOLUTIONS

✓ I will have my vision checked every two years (or annually if needed).

✓ I will report any sudden visual loss, or double vision associated with severe headaches in my temples as an emergency.

✓ I will eat plenty of fruit and vegetables.

✓ I will wear sunglasses in bright sunshine.

Take care of your ... Hearing

In 2015 Age UK reported that an estimated 6.4 million (almost 60 per cent) of people aged 65 and over have hearing loss. Of those, 685,000 are profoundly deaf. Loss affects all sound frequencies, but especially higher ones – making children's and women's voices harder to hear (see www.nhs.uk).

Age Related Hearing Loss (ARHL, formerly called *presbycusis*) affect almost everyone and is due to gradual loss of sound-sensitive cells, nerves, or delicate supporting structures in the tiny hearing organs deep within your ears. Age-related changes sometimes cause unpleasant sounds (tinnitus) or impair the balance organs nearby.

Age-related changes

Age-related hearing loss can cause major disability due to poor communication, which can lead to inactivity and social withdrawal, isolation, depression, loss of fitness, physical and mental ill-health and ultimately preventable death.

The charity Action on Hearing Loss (formerly the Royal National Institute of the Deaf) hosts an online hearing test at www.actiononhearingloss.org. uk. Their research shows that while 1 in 10 adults in the UK would benefit from using a hearing aid, only 1 in 30 actually uses one.

The disinclination to use aids is the main problem for age-related hearing loss. You really needn't feel embarrassed about being hard of hearing. The NHS can provide discrete, easy to manage devices and NHS hearing-aid clinics in your area can troubleshoot problems that arise. If you have poor vision or find the tiny aids difficult, you can be fitted with something more suitable.

CLUES TO WHEN YOUR HEARING LOSS IS WORTH INVESTIGATING:

✓ **People complain you turn the TV up too loud.**

✓ **People complain you don't answer them** when they ask you something and you're turned away or in another room.

✓ **People complain you're shouting at them.**

✓ **You have difficulty hearing conversation**, particularly women's or children's voices, when there's background noise.

If you have recently noticed hearing loss, it is important to exclude uncommon but more serious problems, so do see your GP.

The most important things to consider when you go for a hearing test are: is wax blocking your ears, is your reduced hearing on one or both sides and would you wear a hearing aid if you were offered one?

Wax is common but becomes more of a problem with increasing age because it gets thicker, so blocks the ears more quickly. If it's wax, and hearing improves after clearing it, there's no more to be said. If hearing loss is on both sides and remains after clearing wax it is more likely to be ARHL. But there is little point having further hearing tests UNLESS you are prepared to try using a hearing aid.

One-sided hearing loss (especially with tinnitus or wobbliness on one side) may be due to pressure on your hearing and balance nerve from a tiny tumour. Your GP may recommend hearing tests and a hospital referral to check this out.

Tinnitus (buzzing, humming or ringing in the ears) and **balance problems** also get more common with age. They can be due to disease and need assessment by your GP.

Tinnitus is distressing but distraction techniques can help, it often fades with time and sometimes people just adapt. If it's severe, wearing earphones with 'white noise' can help block it out.

If you have a balance problem please see your GP to establish the cause and get appropriate treatment to reduce the risk of falls. If you have a balance problem when your head moves in certain directions, it may be something called benign positional vertigo (BPV). Your GP may be able to perform the Epley manoeuvre (see www.nhs.uk) to help.

What you can do for your hearing

1. **Take hearing loss seriously**. See your GP: is it ARHL or something else? Wax needs removal before hearing can be assessed.
2. **If ARHL is confirmed**: decide whether you will wear a hearing aid if offered.
3. **If you are ready to try an aid for ARHL**, discuss this with your GP. NHS audiology is done either in hospital (if there is uncertainty about the cause, or other complications) or high street stores with NHS contracts (such as Specsavers).

CLEARING EARWAX THE SAFE WAY

DO NOT poke a cotton bud, a hairgrip or similar into your ear – you may damage your eardrum. Drop or spray sodium bicarbonate solution or olive oil in the affected ear(s) about three times daily for 10 days, and follow your pharmacist's instructions. See your practice nurse if the wax does not come out.

Red flags

- **Sudden hearing loss** needs medical assessment. There may be a simple explanation, but occasionally a more serious problem needs sorting.

- **Gradual onset of one-sided hearing loss**, especially with one-sided tinnitus and/or one-sided balance problems, needs medical assessment ASAP. It may be wax, but it may be a red flag for a small, treatable tumour of your hearing and balance nerve.
- **Ear pain or earache** is not an age-related problem and often occurs with a heavy head cold. Steam inhalations, clearing catarrh, and ibuprofen (if safe for you) can help. If it persists for more than a day or two (at any age), discuss it with your pharmacist or GP.

RESOLUTIONS

✓ I will take hearing loss seriously.

✓ I won't stick anything in my ear.

Take care of your ... Hair

By the time you are 60 your hair will usually be less abundant and colourful than it was in your 20s. How you take care of it depends on what matters to your self-image and self-esteem. For some people, it's essential to pursue options for restoring loss of hair colour or quantity; for others, it's something they accept and adapt to.

Age-related changes

Age-related changes to your crowning glory start well before your 50s, and loss of hair colour is usually the first (we still don't understand why and no, it's NOT been proved it's stress).

There are **two** main types of age-related hair loss: one hormone-sensitive, the other not. By aged 50, fifty per cent of men have some hair loss on top of their head – **hormone sensitive** male-pattern baldness. A similar process, though less well understood, can affect some women too – female-pattern hair loss. It is usually much less extensive than in men, more concentrated along the hair parting and rarely affecting the whole top.

It doesn't affect everyone, but in both sexes when it does, it's due to your genetically determined sensitivity to circulating androgen hormones (testosterone and similar). If you're very sensitive, hair loss can start early in adult life and continue with time. Women continue to produce low levels of androgens after their menopause, which is why female pattern hair loss can continue into the 50s and 60s if they are sensitive – but the role of lower post-menopausal oestrogen levels is not clear. Increased growth of facial hair (facial hirsutism), which is also androgen sensitive, may occur either with female pattern hair loss or alone.

A **second** type of age-related hair loss not linked to hormone sensitivity can occur in our 60s and beyond, causing more diffuse thinning over the whole head.

Changes to hair with disease and its treatment

Most problems affecting our hair are due to skin problems on our scalp. The most common is dandruff. There is excellent advice at NHS Choices (www.nhs.net) on this and other problems like eczema and psoriasis.

Less commonly, conditions can affect hair texture (an underactive thyroid), or loss (alopecia) due to a variety of problems unrelated to age. Occasionally, if natural hair colour remains, an immune related problem (vitiligo) can cause whitened patches. In women, excess facial hair growth (sometimes called facial hirsutism) can cause distress and, if it is **very** extensive, it is a good idea to check with your doctor that there is no underlying problem with your hormones or metabolic health.

Chemotherapy-related hair loss is something people often dread and is entirely dependent on which drugs are used in the chemotherapy regime. This drug-induced total baldness (anagen effluvium) is *almost always* temporary.

Depending on the drugs used, it may be relevant to discuss wearing cold caps during chemotherapy to reduce the circulation of drugs to the scalp and so reduce hair loss. There are pros and cons. You may have to stay in hospital longer if you have cold cap treatment. Some patients choose to wear a wig. Preparing one in advance is good advice, as you do not know how you will feel until it occurs. Others shave their remaining hair: a fashion and, increasingly, an image statement. Some use headscarves, turbans, hats and caps.

What you can do for your hair

There are no set rules. Over- or under-washing can make the scalp over-dry or leave it over-oily. Dyes and other hair products can irritate – and should be avoided if they do. Blow-drying can make hair brittle and break, and combing or brushing after washing without using conditioner can pull out remaining hair from the roots: worth avoiding if your hair has thinned.

If you look after small children, including your grandchildren, nits are common. If they need treatment, so do you.

The NHS does not usually make cosmetic procedures or medicines for hair loss available given its resources. So for most people treatment for loss (apart from chemotherapy related), or excessive hair, has to be private or over-the-counter.

1. For top of the head, age-related hair loss in men or women:

- **Protect the top of your head from the sun**. The scalp is very exposed and pre-cancerous skin changes are common. Wear a hat or scarf.
- **Wigs** or **toupees**.
- **Minoxidil** ONLY treats age-related hair loss due to testosterone sensitivity. You can buy it as a 5 per cent mousse for once daily application. It isn't always effective and has potential side effects – please discuss it with your pharmacist FIRST. Any re-growth wears off when you stop using it.
- **Hair transplants** – typically in men (small sections of hair from the back of the head are transplanted to the top). **This can go wrong** – so think carefully before you go ahead.

2. For the treatment for excessive hair:

- **Depilatory creams**.
- **Electrolysis**.
- **Medicated cream**, containing eflornithine (Vaniqa). It is not routinely available on prescription, and can cause side effects.
- **Laser treatment**, but this only works on dark pigmented hair and not white or grey – so is of limited use.

RESOLUTION

✓ I will ask myself what really matters to me about my hair.

Take care of your ... Skin

Lines, wrinkles and greying hair are usually the first clues that we are getting older. They start to happen years before we reach our 60s. We notice the changes because they occur on our face, head and hands, which we see in the mirror every day. But if we compare the skin on our face and hands with that on our tummy or inner thighs, where it is less exposed to sunlight, it is noticeably smoother and sometimes wrinkle-free.

Age-related changes

Changes are not uniform over the body and vary between people too, even on parts that are exposed. Smokers often have more noticeable changes, as do people in outdoor occupations or those who have holidayed in the sun with little protection from its rays. 'Weathered skin' is a good description of much of the change we see. Age-related skin changes come from within too. Skin loses significant elastin in its deeper layer, so it doesn't spring back so quickly when it's folded, pressed or creased. It becomes drier and less flexible, as less natural oil is produced, predisposing it to irritation and infection. Exposure to sunlight and the elements accentuates these problems.

We want the benefits of sun exposure but not its harms. Sunlight helps the skin make vitamin D and makes us warm and relaxed, lifting our mood. It is a real 'feel-good factor'. During the summer in the UK, 10–15 minutes exposure to bright sunlight daily (a little more with dark skin), avoiding high sun which will burn, produces sufficient vitamin D and should be adequate up to age 65 if you have a healthy balanced diet. (Over 65 years, a supplement of 10 micrograms is recommended.) In the winter, you'll need more from your diet (oily fish twice a week, eggs, vitamin D fortified breakfast cereals – check on the packet – or a supplement), as insufficient UV light is available for skin to make vitamin D, so your body uses its stores.

The problem is that sunlight is a major factor causing skin cancers – especially melanoma (cancerous moles), and a variety of other pre-cancerous skin changes.

What you can do for your skin

It's all about the four Ps: Prevention, Protection, Picking things up early and Promptly treating problems you find. Here are the rules for taking care of your skin:

1. **Protect your exposed parts from too much sunlight** – use at least a factor 15 sunscreen that **also** has a star rating that confirms protection against UVA as well as UVB light, as both contribute to skin cancer. Cover up in the sun: wear a wide-brimmed hat, shades and a cotton cover over your body.
2. **Ensure you get enough vitamin D** from your diet (see above, and NHS Choices) and a supplement if needed.

3. **Moisturise your skin** – including the hidden bits. Use a cream daily (e.g. aqueous cream) and a greasy moisturiser weekly (or mix in some Vaseline or similar white soft paraffin grease from the supermarket or pharmacy to your aqueous routine), but more often if your skin is very dry.

4. **Regularly check for new moles and changes** in those you have, enlist the help of partners or close friends if needed. Use mirrors.

5. **Wash regularly and DRY SCRUPULOUSLY BUT GENTLY in the deep recesses** where moisture, sweat, urine and faeces collect and feed yeasts and bacteria.

Red flags

- A **mole** that's changed in **any** way.
- A **skin ulcer**, anywhere, that's open and won't heal.
- A **horny, hard patch of skin** that's getting bigger, in a place you wouldn't expect. Most of us get hard skin over a pressure point: for example at the back of our heel, over a bunion or a corn on a rubbed toe. But we're talking about odd, new patches where you don't expect them.
- **Cracks and skin infections between the toes**, especially if you're diabetic, when this needs URGENT treatment.
- A skin problem that you have been diagnosed with (for example **eczema** or **psoriasis**) that's getting out of control.

RESOLUTIONS

✓ I will use sun protection and a hat in the sunshine.

✓ I will check out changing moles promptly.

✓ I will treat foot infections promptly, and urgently if I have diabetes.

✓ I will moisturise regularly: a creamy one daily and a greasy one weekly – or more.

Every Breath You Take, Every Beat you Make

Now, lets talk about your lungs and your heart.

Take care of your ... Lungs

Your lungs provide the oxygen you need moment by moment, so they need your care.

Age-related changes

Puffing power declines a bit year by year. But it's a gentle drop until very old age. Ageing causes a slight reduction of volume into which the lungs can expand, and a small reduction in the strength of breathing muscles and elasticity of connective tissues that allow the lungs to expand and contract.

Your lungs will reflect your past exposure to environmental toxins: passive smoking and air pollution, for example. The causes may have gone but traces of their effects may remain. The Clean Air Act was passed in 1956, so us 60-somethings were only exposed as baby baby-boomers and escaped the years of toxic damage our older brothers and sisters were exposed to.

If you smoke, the bad news is that your breathing efficiency will deteriorate at a much greater rate, leaving you breathless even with slight exertion or at rest. You are also likely to have serious and frequent chest infections, which can contribute to more chronic lung problems and even heart failure.

The good news is that even if you have smoked for most of your life, you can put the brake on your deteriorating lung function if you stop now.

What you can do for your lungs

If you smoke, the first and most important thing to do is to **STOP, NOW!**

This will remove the factors leading to rapid loss of lung function. You won't be able to reverse all the historical damage, but you will be able to slow the rate of further deterioration, and improve chest problems like chronic bronchitis (a form of 'chronic obstructive airways disease', or COPD). Stopping smoking is rather like 'closing the fitness gap' for the lungs. It can make all the difference to your well-being now, and to your health and independence in the future.

YOU *CAN* STOP SMOKING

There is no safe level of smoking – so stop completely, if you can. And here's some good news if you haven't:

✓ **You can do it**. Many people in their 50s and 60s HAVE quit smoking. For once, we baby-boomers can lay claim to fame at 60 as we have the lowest rate of smoking in the UK. If your peers can quit, there's a good chance you can.

✓ **It's never too late**. However long you've smoked you **can** quit – it's **worth** it.

✓ **Just *try* stopping. If you can't, then try again**. The more you try the more likely you are to succeed.

✓ **Don't wait**. Often people are only jet propelled into quitting when a serious medical event, like a heart attack, stroke or cancer, happens to them, or someone they love. Why put yourself through that?

Top tips to help you stop smoking

1. **If you smoke 10 or more cigarettes a day think about getting help** from your pharmacist or GP practice. Or try the NHS smoke-free website www.nhs.uk/smokefree, or patient.co.uk

2. **Try nicotine replacement therapy** (NRT) first. Evidence suggests that NRT, which you gradually reduce, can help manage chemical withdrawal while you start changing your smoking-related behaviour.

3. Choose a **QUIT DATE** (your birthday, the New Year, or the due date of a new grandchild). Throw out all the paraphernalia of smoking – cigarettes, ashtrays, lighters and so on – the night before you start.

4. **Get a money box**. The night before your quit date, put the amount you'd spend on cigarettes in a day in it. Add to it daily, it's what you would have spent on cigarettes – hear that rattle!

5. **Get exercising**. Put in a positive fitness factor while you remove a negative harm. It can help reduce weight gain, a common, temporary behavioural consequence of over-eating when you first stop smoking.

There has been a rapid rise in the use of e-cigarettes and Public Health England has now approved them to help even more people quit. But it is wise to be cautious about any additional chemicals you use.

Other things you can do to look after your lungs

- **Get your annual flu vaccination** (if appropriate for you, see Chapter 9).
- **Get walking**, and do your chest, core and upper limb girdle strengthening exercises (see page 37–40).
- **Look after asthma**. Make sure you understand how and when to use your inhalers. If you have weak hands, ask your pharmacist, practice nurse or GP for a simple aid to help you.
- **Keep your posture upright**.
- **Practise mindful breathing**.

Red flags

- **If you cough up blood** and there's no obvious reason (like having had a nosebleed, or a heavy cold), see your GP.
- **If you have a NEW unexplained, persistent cough (which lasts for more than 3–4 weeks)** see your GP, especially if you've ever smoked heavily. lung cancer needs excluding.
- **If your asthma is uncontrollable**, see your GP (but first check your inhalers aren't out of date).
- **If you are suddenly breathless** with exertion or at rest, especially if you have chest pain and a new cough, see your GP urgently.

RESOLUTIONS

✓ If I smoke I will try to quit – and keep trying.

✓ I will have my annual flu vaccination, if needed.

✓ If I cough up blood without any signs of a cold, sinusitis or a nosebleed, I will see my GP.

Take care of your ... Heart and circulation

The stunning statistic is that **physical activity alone reduces your risk of heart disease by over 40 per cent** (see page 24). You can also help by reducing avoidable stress, losing any excess weight, eating a Mediterranean-style diet, stopping smoking and managing high blood pressure. Carefully considering taking a statin medication – to reduce a high risk of heart disease, or manage it better if you have it – is very important too.

Your heart is a muscular organ. Its rate is governed by a natural pacemaker and regulated by your activity, emotions and any medication that slows or quickens it.

It can even be restarted if it stops prematurely as long as someone skilled in CPR (cardiopulmonary resuscitation) is on hand to help or a defibrillator is available. Many public places now have defibrillators, which are clearly marked and simple to use in an emergency. They tell you what to do as you go along – even if you've never been trained – and this can save someone's life.

Thankfully, modern treatment of heart attacks and severe angina has improved survival rates. Stents (tiny tubes to open blocked vessels) increase blood flow immediately. Medication (to lower heart rate, improve its function, lower unhelpful cholesterol and thin the blood) helps too. The combination of better medication and a healthier lifestyle reduces recurrence – a good example of secondary prevention (see Chapter 1).

Many survivors of a heart attack feel healthier than before, because they've had a 'wake-up call'. They stop smoking, get more active, reduce excess weight and lower their unhelpful LDL cholesterol. **Statin medication and aspirin** (or similar drugs) are strongly recommended for anyone after a heart attack or angina. But despite medical advances, cardiovascular diseases are still the leading cause of death in people over 65 in the UK.

TO TAKE OR NOT TO TAKE STATINS – THAT IS THE QUESTION

The fact is that statins lower cholesterol levels in most people – specifically, the bad LDL cholesterol, which contributes to clogged arteries and heart attacks. Statins will always be recommended after a heart attack. But they also reduce the risk of a first heart attack (your Q-risk, especially if it is high, e.g. a one in five chance or more over 10 years).

However, they can have side effects: mild bloating, liver irritation and occasionally muscle inflammation. Though these will all settle on stopping statins, weighing their significant benefit against possible harm is important, especially if your Q-risk is low. More recent studies show a small increased risk of type 2 diabetes, but experts think this is in people about to get it anyway. Even then, they still reduce the overall risk of heart attack.

But whatever your Q-risk, you can reduce it and reduce the risk of type 2 diabetes by losing excess weight, getting more active, eating a Mediterranean diet, stopping smoking and controlling high blood pressure. Doing this for 6 months might reduce your Q-risk significantly. So you could try this before starting statins.

If your risk remains high despite your efforts, statins are there to help. The National Institute for Health and Care (NICE) now recommends a statin even at the lower risk of a one in ten chance of heart attack over 10 years, but you have to weigh it up. A low dose statin pill IS available over the counter, so the choice is yours. Do discuss it with your pharmacist and GP, as you need a blood test to check your liver before and after starting.

Age-related changes

Like any muscle, your heart loses a little power with age and its *maximum possible rate* decreases slightly year by year. But the main age related changes are due to two processes. Firstly, loss of fitness. Inactivity makes heart muscle lose power rapidly (as with any muscle) so it gets less efficient, and you get breathless and tire more quickly with exercise. Secondly, clogging up of the arteries (*atherosclerosis*) due to an unhealthy lifestyle and other risk factors (see page 76). Atherosclerosis reduces blood supply to the heart itself (*coronary artery disease*), the brain (*cerebrovascular disease*) and the rest of the body (*peripheral vascular disease*).

Coronary artery disease can lead to a number of different health problems:

1. Angina and heart attacks
The difference between angina and a heart attack is that in the former a coronary artery is narrow but not blocked off, whereas in the latter it is.

Angina is chest pain during exertion but not at rest. A heart attack is chest pain even at rest, or which persists even if you do. **Chest pain at rest is a big red flag for a suspected heart attack. It should prompt a 999 (or 112 on your mobile) call to get you to hospital quickly**.

2. Irregular pulse
Atrial fibrillation (AF) is an irregular heartbeat and major risk factor for blood clots, which cause stroke and block leg arteries. When rapid, it can cause heart failure. This is why it's important to report an irregular pulse. If it's AF, blood-thinning treatment (not aspirin) is needed to reduce the risk of stroke and unnecessary loss of limb.

3. Heart failure
This is important to take seriously, and can cause sudden or recent onset of breathlessness with minimal exertion. The combination of coronary heart disease with chronic lung disease is a potent cause of preventable heart failure, mainly due to smoking.

Cerebrovascular disease reduces the blood supply to the brain, and is also caused by atherosclerosis (see page 109). **Peripheral vascular disease** narrows arteries to the other organs and to the limbs. Narrowed leg arteries cause leg muscle pain on exercise, which subsides on resting, called 'intermittent claudication'. Impotence (or erectile dysfunction, see page 142) can be a sign of peripheral vascular disease and an early warning of coronary artery disease even before angina. So if you are impotent, check it out even if you're not sexually active. It could be an important red flag.

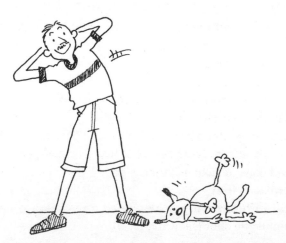

DO YOU HAVE RISK FACTORS FOR HEART DISEASE?

The main risk factors for heart and vascular disease are an unhealthy lifestyle (inactivity, smoking, excess weight), high blood pressure (hypertension), raised LDL cholesterol and blood sugar (metabolic syndrome), diabetes and a family history (even with a healthy lifestyle). If in doubt – check it out. The NHS runs free health checks for people aged 40–74, and your cholesterol is tested. If you haven't had one, then ask for it. If you're a man aged 65 or more, you will be invited for a painless ultrasound scan, to exclude abdominal aortic aneurysm. It is more common in men, and if present, can occasionally burst or leak, causing rapid collapse and death.

What you can do for your heart

- **Stop smoking**.
- **Get active and stay active**: keep up your two and a half hours of slightly puffy activity a week and WALK EVERYWERE YOU CAN!
- **Adopt a Mediterranean diet**: lower your unhelpful LDL cholesterol and reduce sugar, especially sugary drinks (see page 84).
- **Lose excess weight**: find and keep your healthy weight.
- **Bust stress**: it really does contribute to heart disease (and many other illnesses too). Take it seriously and take action: de-stress, practise mindfulness, look at your schedule and get help for underlying problems (see page 62–70).
- **Keep your blood pressure under control**: by reducing excess weight, stress, excess alcohol and salt. **Take your blood-pressure medication regularly**. Report any side effects to your GP, so they can be managed. A reduction of as little as 5mm of mercury pressure significantly reduces your stroke risk.
- **Statins and aspirin (or a similar drug)** are strongly recommended after a heart attack or angina, if they don't cause you serious side effects (see page 108–109). However, please discuss the pros and cons of taking statins if your Q-risk is raised with your GP or pharmacist **first**.
- **Prevent influenza**: if you have heart disease, make sure you have your annual flu shot (see Chapter 9).

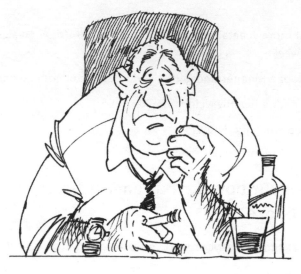

Red flags

- **Sudden chest pain at rest** or that continues even if you do rest, or the **sudden development of a white, painful leg** suggests a heart attack or a blocked leg artery. **Both need 999**. You need to go to hospital immediately.
- **Chest pain, cramping leg muscle pain, or recent onset of severe breathlessness** related to exertion might be angina, intermittent claudication or heart failure. See your GP.
- **An irregular pulse**. Please see your GP to rule out atrial fibrillation.
- **Unexplained blackouts** – may be due to your heart rate slowing. See your GP.
- **If you develop a painful, swollen, tender calf especially** after a long flight, coach or car journey, a deep vein thrombosis (DVT) needs ruling out. Hormone replacement therapy increases your risk. Please see your GP.

RESOLUTIONS

✓ I will do at least 30 minutes of sweaty, puffy activity daily in bits or chunks.

✓ I will get my blood pressure checked, reduce it if high and reduce salt intake.

✓ I will eat more vegetables and fruit, and oily fish (or equivalent) twice a week.

✓ I will adopt a Mediterranean diet and use olive oil for cooking

✓ I will aim for a healthy weight and keep it.

✓ I will stop smoking, NOW!

Your bite, your bowel, your energy balance and your booze

Now it's time to talk about your teeth, your digestive tract and your liver.

Taking care of your ... Teeth and gums

Well, what can you expect of your teeth after 60-odd years of unhelpful lifestyle, contact with sugar and other odds and ends of food that provide a marvellous culture medium for bacteria?

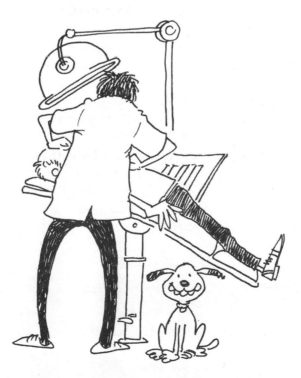

Age-related changes

The main problem is, of course, the plaque at the junction of your teeth and gums, which causes gum inflammation and infection making them bleed and finally shrink away from their normal protective place adherent to the base of the tooth. This exposes the dentine, which sits below normal gum level and which bacteria can attack easily, helping them spread further onto the surface enamel of the tooth which they eat away too, helped by acids from fruit and other foods.

If you use mouthwash, avoid the ones containing alcohol, as they increase the risk of mouth cancer. Warm salt water is all you need, but if you have a sore throat, the brief use of antiseptic mouthwash for a clean and a gargle is fine.

What you can do for your teeth

- **Don't miss your regular dental checks**. Your dentist is highly trained, and looks for signs of mouth (oral) disease including cancer, as well as evidence of tooth decay, infections, and more serious dental problems.
- **Don't delay**. If you've got a painful tooth, see your dentist before you develop an abscess. It is one of the worst pains you can have.

SEVEN TOP TIPS FOR HEALTHY TEETH AND GUMS

1. **Reduce the sugar in your diet** and don't suck sugary sweets.

2. The **mix of sugar and acid in cola drinks can dissolve the enamel** quickly.

3. **Brush for 2 minutes twice daily**. Don't use a hard brush, and use a circular movement (or an electric toothbrush if you prefer) so you don't wear down the enamel. If the gum bleeds, continue brushing till it stops, to clear plaque.

4. **Floss daily**, and **use a toothpaste containing flouride**. Choose one for sensitive teeth if it's pain that's putting you off brushing – is this a reminder to see your dentist?

5. **Neutralise acid foods** you've eaten (an apple, for example) with an alkali, like milk or cheese.

6. **If you have dentures,** brush them twice daily, as well as sterilising them.

7. **Visit the hygienist** and the dentist regularly.

Red flags

- **Bleeding gums despite good tooth brushing** and oral hygiene – see your GP.
- **Pain in your tooth/jaw,** especially if swollen and tender – see your dentist.
- **If you are starting bone-protection medication** (*bisphosphonates*), see your dentist to get planned dental treatment completed before starting the medication, which can occasionally complicate dental surgery.

RESOLUTIONS

✓ I will brush my teeth gently for 2 minutes or longer twice daily, until any bleeding stops. I will floss every day.

✓ If my gums continue to bleed after brushing my teeth well after a couple of days I will see my dentist or doctor.

✓ I will not drink sugary drinks or suck sweets.

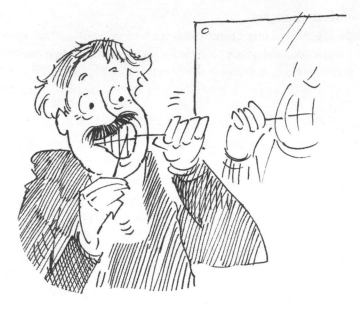

Take care of your ... Digestion and liver

Your digestive tract extends from your mouth to your anus, and includes your liver and pancreas (important for your metabolic health, see page 75). They produce digestive juices – bile from your liver (collecting in your gall bladder), and enzymes from your pancreas (which digest fat). The liver breaks down alcohol and is affected by it.

Your gut is a muscular tube, propelling food along its length, and fibre is critical to its smooth function. It digests and absorbs most of your food and drink, apart from the fibre. Its walls contain specialised immune tissue, important for your health. Occasionally, this causes problems, for example when people with coeliac disease (a sensitivity to the wheat protein gluten) eat products containing it.

What can go wrong? Well, a spectrum of activity, from constipation to windy diarrhoea called irritable bowel syndrome. IBS is not a disease but an *awareness* of over- or under-stimulation of the bowel, which can cause troublesome symptoms at any age.

Your liver processes all the products of digestion it receives from your bowel. If you consume more than you need, excess calories are converted to fat. We saw in the last chapter how this leads to excess weight, central fat and metabolic ill health. Some excess fat gets stored in the liver itself – which is bad for its health (see page 119).

Age-related changes

The slight age-related loss of muscle power and connective tissue elasticity affects the gut too, and tends to slow it down – making constipation more likely. You may bring conditions with you into your 60s: acid reflux and indigestion are common, especially with excess weight, smoking and excess alcohol.

Constipation and irritable bowel syndrome are common too, and can overlap, but new onset persistent irritable bowel symptoms or persistent change in bowel pattern are unusual in your 60s and red flags to check out (see page 122). More commonly, constipation is due to inadequate dietary fibre, inactivity and sometimes side effects of codeine-based painkillers: all of which slows the gut, allowing more water to be absorbed. This forms hard stool: which IS constipation.

With constipation and straining come piles (or haemorrhoids): little swellings in the veins of the anus, that can be painful for a few days, and can sometimes bleed when you do a poo. You can get soothing cream (like Anusol) from your pharmacist, but the main treatment is to tackle the constipation so you don't strain. However, if you have bleeding from your bottom and it's new, please see your GP to exclude bowel cancer.

FARTS AND FOOD

We all make wind, some more than others. We can control it by tightening the muscles around our back passage, though not always successfully. Pelvic floor exercises can help (see page 137–138).

It's not often that farts indicate disease, but occasionally so, for example if you've picked up a gut parasite, like giardia, on your travels abroad. But mostly wind and farts are due to a combination of what we eat and the unique mix of bacteria that live in our large bowel. Many bacteria can digest fibre that we can't. They ferment it, releasing a variety of harmless but interesting smells in the process. If you have a problem with wind, experiment with different types and combinations of fibre (see page 119). If you can't sort it, you could ask your GP about referral to a dietician.

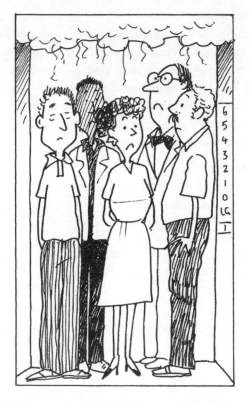

Most age-related changes in the digestive tract and liver are age-related effects of other factors, particularly dietary habits. With bowel cancer, there are important genetic factors too, and liver problems may be compounded by age-related consequences of infection with the hepatitis viruses. However, the main changes are as follows:

1. Diverticular changes (*diverticulosis*)
This is when tiny pouches of gut lining get forced through weak points in the bowel wall. The biggest cause is constipation, due to insufficient dietary fibre (low-residue food), that doesn't give the bowel wall muscles anything to work on. They get weaker and less effective at propelling food along. Digested food stays in the colon longer, making the faeces hard and more difficult to propel, blocking the bowel.

Diverticular 'pouches' may not cause any problems. But, like your appendix, they can get infected and inflamed (typically causing pain on the left side of your lower tummy), or bleed and occasionally burst. Burst bowel, wherever it happens, is always dangerous. So diverticulosis is best avoided by treating constipation.

2. Fatty liver change

This is when fat gets deposited throughout the substance of the liver where it normally isn't found. It causes inflammation, scarring and eventually cirrhosis, which leads to liver cancer and other problems. Obesity – now so common in our 60s – is the leading cause of fatty liver change and cirrhosis, and has overtaken alcohol as a cause of liver disease. But alcohol is calorie-rich, so is a double dose of liver harm, contributing to fatty liver by excess calories, as well as toxic effects.

3. Digestive tract cancers

Bowel cancer is one of the commonest cancers in the UK. There is good information at the NHS Choices website (www.nhs.uk). The important risk factors are alcohol, which increases the risk of all bowel cancers (even at 'safe levels'), smoking, eating lots of red meat and nitrate-preserved processed meats, like sausages and ham, which combine with stomach acid to increase the risk of stomach cancer.

PROTECT YOUR BOWEL WITH FIBRE

You can prevent constipation, diverticulosis and piles by ensuring that you have sufficient fibre (and fluid) in your diet. Fibre can help your bowel function better, and contributes to your metabolic health.

There are two types of fibre. Soluble fibre absorbs water, so softens and bulks the faeces – speeding bowel movement and reducing the time digested food stays in the gut. This, and its property of binding some digested fats and sugars, leads to reductions in LDL cholesterol and blood sugar. It is found in grains, fruits, roots and golden linseed (see www.nhs.uk), which you can sprinkle on food but is best avoided if you have diarrhoea.

Insoluble fibre is found in bran, many nuts and seeds, cereals and wholemeal products. It gives the bowel muscle something solid to work against, keeping it strong and active. Wholegrains are good sources of soluble and insoluble fibre – which work best when in combination.

You may need to experiment with the amount and balance. On average, most adults need around 30g (just over an ounce) of total fibre daily, of which a small amount (about 3g) is best as the soluble sort. You can usually find details on cereal packets.

A family history of bowel cancer increases your risk. If you have had a parent or sibling with multiple colon polyps (little growths) called polyposis, you should have regular colonoscopies, as you will be at increased risk of polyps too, which can occasionally turn cancerous.

What you can do for your digestion and liver

Look in the box above about fibre first, then have a look at the following seven suggestions:

1. **Manage constipation**: over 1 in 7 of all adults suffer from constipation, and it gets more common as we get older. Drink more water, increase your fibre or see your GP if you can't solve the problem.
2. **Don't strain**: it aggravates diverticula, piles, prolapses and stress incontinence (see page 152).
3. **Avoid excess calories**: especially sugary ones from drinks.
4. **Reduce red meats and nitrite preserved (cured) meats** (salamis, hams etc).
5. **All alcohol has risk** but it's a balance – always keep within safe limits.
6. **Stop smoking**.
7. **Check your hepatitis immunity if you are,** or have been, at risk (see below).
8. **Consider eating plain live yogurt** after antibiotics or an episode of acute, infective diarrhoea. It can replace your bowel's helpful lactobacillus bacteria.

KEEPING YOUR ALCOHOL IN SAFE LIMITS

Alcohol, in moderation, is enjoyed by most people. It is not risk-free, but acceptably safe if you keep within the recommended maximum units, spread through the week.

One alcohol unit is the equivalent of:

✓ 25mls (a single measure) of whisky (ABV = 40%).

✓ One third of a pint of beer (ABV = 5–6%).

✓ Half a standard 175ml glass (87mls) of red, rose or white wine (ABV = 12%), but less than that (75mls) if the ABV is 13.5%, which is now very common.

(ABV is the alcohol by volume.)

The recommendations for safe limits are:

✓ **21 units maximum per week for men**.

✓ **14 units maximum per week for women**.

✓ **Maximum** daily: **3–4 units for men**, or **2–3 units for women** – but clearly not every day, as this would exceed the weekly limit.

✓ **Minimum** weekly: **three alcohol-free days**, but ideally four.

✓ **NO ALCOHOL** if you're going to drive or do any job requiring your judgement. Avoid lunchtime drinking if you need to concentrate in the afternoon.

A bottle of wine (ABV 13.5) has 10 units of alcohol, and if equally shared between two people gives each more than their ideal daily intake. Remember, one small glass of wine in a pub (175 ml) will be around 2 units (depending on the ABV of the wine). Most pubs only serve larger glasses – which would make 'just one' glass of wine exceed your daily limit.

If you're drinking more because your mood is low, or you have to drink first thing in the morning, you need help urgently. Your GP, Alcoholics Anonymous (AA) and local alcohol support services can provide it. But you need to take the first step. Don't store up your problems; ask for help, now!

Have a blood test for **hepatitis B** and **C** if you have a high risk of infection: past intravenous drug use (especially if you shared needles), or unprotected sex with different partners. This is a common story among baby-boomers so you may have been at risk. Your surgery can offer advice and counselling, but the sooner you are diagnosed the better.

- **If you are hepatitis C or hepatitis B** (hep C or B) **positive**: you should seek medical advice and avoid alcohol altogether.
- **If you are hepatitis B negative and still at risk**, get a hep B vaccination. As yet there is NO hep C vaccination: though vaccines are being developed and assessed in research trials.

Red flags

- **If there's blood in your poo for a week or two, it may be cancer** and the earlier it's picked up and treated, the better the outcome. See your GP ASAP.
- **Frequent, loose bloody poo**, with pain in your tummy and when you go to the loo, may be **inflammatory bowel disease or IBD** (for example, ulcerative colitis or Crohn's disease). This is **not** to be confused with irritable bowel syndrome (IBS), which is much less serious. See your GP ASAP.
- **Pain in your tummy, indigestion that doesn't settle, pain or difficulty with swallowing**, especially if new, not going away or getting worse. See your GP ASAP – the same day if the pain is severe.
- **If you feel a lump in your tummy**: see your GP ASAP.
- **Any change in bowel habits**: new constipation, diarrhoea, or a fluctuating pattern persisting for more than two weeks, see your GP ASAP to rule out cancer.
- **Feeling unusually bloated in your lower tummy if you're a woman**: if this is new to you and persists more than a month **don't** assume it's irritable bowel. Ovarian cysts, occasionally cancerous, need ruling out ASAP.
- **Unexplained continuing weight loss**, when you're not trying to lose it – go and see your GP ASAP.

Fibre and inflammatory bowel disease (IBD)

If you have ulcerative colitis or Crohn's (both types of IBD) you should always get personalised dietary advice from your consultant or dietician, including about fibre. You will almost always be advised to AVOID insoluble fibre especially fruit skins, pips and seeds, if you have a flare of your condition. Usually, flares of ulcerative colitis will be helped by a very low fibre diet.

RESOLUTIONS

✓ I will eat a Mediterranean diet with daily vegetables and fruit and oily fish twice a week.

✓ I will ensure I eat enough fibre to keep my bowel active.

✓ If I drink alcohol I will keep it within safe limits.

✓ I will reduce red meat in my diet, and minimise processed, preserved meats.

✓ I will report any blood in my poo, lump in my tummy, or persistent change in bowel habit to my GP.

✓ I will drink more water if I'm drinking less than 6–8 glasses a day.

Every move you make, every step you take

Down, down we go to your muscles and bones, joints, spine and feet.

Take care of your ... Muscles

Muscles are at the heart of your health. To keep them powerful you need to keep them active. Use them or lose them. Your skeletal muscles are key to your strength, power and endurance (see Chapter 2). When they're strong, they correct wobbles more rapidly – preventing falls. And having more muscle to fat, especially around your middle, is a component of fitness (see Chapter 4).

Age-related changes

We covered the most important things in Chapter 1. You may want to flip back to remind yourself (see page 16).

What you can do for your muscles

A study of cyclists aged 55–79 who had continued active cycling throughout their adult life, found hardly any age-related difference in muscle power. By keeping active they had closed their fitness gap. So remember that your daily routine of 10 minutes stretching and strengthening, with as much walking as you can, will work wonders for your muscle (and mental) health.

If you're a woman in your 60s, you'll need even more exercise as you get older, to compensate for age-related change and lower post menopausal oestrogen. It has dropped more dramatically than the gradual age-related fall in testosterone in men. T'ai chi is great for building muscle (and bone) strength – especially if you keep it going. To prevent muscle overstrain don't overdo the recommended repetitions, and build up your strength gradually.

Red flags

If you have a sprain or minor muscle injury, don't faff, use First Aid First (FAF) to limit bruising and swelling. The acronym PRICE is your guide – **P**rotect from further injury, **R**est the injured muscle, **I**ce it (a bag of frozen peas wrapped in a tea-towel), **C**ompression (a bandage or compression tube) and **E**levation (keeping it raised up to reduce blood flow). You will need to rest the affected muscles for a few days.

Anti-inflammatories (like ibuprofen) work partly by reducing the blood flow to inflamed areas, so if they're safe for you to use, they can help sprains and strains, ideally as a 'rub-in' or spray. But for the same reason, they may NOT be best for injuries that need good blood flow to get repaired. So please check safety issues in either case with your pharmacist.

- **More significant pain, bruising and swelling?** See your practice nurse or GP. Ask advice on when to resume gentle exercise as appropriate, so the muscles don't become weak, or the joints stiff.
- **If pain, swelling and tenderness is very severe**, or you suspect that the muscle or ligament is completely torn, see your GP or go to A&E.
- **Repetitive strain injury (RSI) is very unlikely with 10 minutes or so of the exercises described in this book.** But it is common around the wrist after intensive painting, cleaning the windows or using your laptop. **RICE** is useful, but a wrist splint and rub-in anti-inflammatory can help – please ask your pharmacist.
- **Painful stiffness of your neck and shoulders which is new and persists**, especially if you're a woman in your later 60s, may be more serious inflammation (*polymyalgia*). It is often worse in the morning. You need to see your doctor.
- **Muscle wasting for no obvious reason** needs medical advice.
- **Persistent muscle swelling** that's not an injury is unusual. Please see your GP.

RESOLUTIONS

✓ I will do my upper limb strengthening exercises (see page 37) daily.

✓ I will do my lower limb strengthening (see page 40–44) daily too, if I am female.

✓ I will walk more, and more briskly.

✓ I will remember PRICE for minor injuries.

Taking care of your ... Bones

Your bones need to be strong and rigid so that your muscles can move the joints rather than bend the bones themselves. Because adult bones aren't bendy they can break if the forces on them are too great or if they are too weak to withstand them. So bone care is about keeping your bones strong and, and even more importantly, preventing falls, which might break them.

Age-related changes

Bone thins with age due to loss of bone mass, or density. Bone is living tissue, in constant turnover. It is estimated that our skeleton turns over and replenishes itself fully about once in seven years. After the peak in our early 30s, the breaking-down processes have a slight edge, so there is net bone loss year by year. The rate of loss due to age alone is small, but if you're a woman it is exaggerated by your lower post-menopausal oestrogen levels.

Special DEXA scans are used to measure bone density. If bones are significantly less dense than normal it's called *osteopenia*, but if more severely so, *osteoporosis*.

The main factors causing bone loss are the usual culprits:

- **Inactivity** and bed rest.
- **Hormone loss** (gradual in men, more dramatic in women after their menopause).
- **Smoking** and **excess alcohol**.
- **Lack of vitamin D** (quite common, as most of us don't get enough sunshine during the winter months) **and lack of calcium** (less common with a healthy, balanced diet).
- **Diseases**, especially an overactive thyroid, and any disease that reduces your activity.
- **Some medications**, most importantly steroids.
- **Family history**. If you have a strong family history of osteoporosis, ensure you work hard to counteract your increased risk of bone thinning.
- Being severely **underweight**.

Even a couple of days in bed has detectable effects. A good motto for bed and bones is 'bed is good for sleep and sex, but not much else'. This is one of the *many* reasons why, nowadays, bed rest for most medical illnesses is as brief as possible.

Brisk walking, jogging, dancing or skipping, for instance, sends shock waves through our weight-bearing bones. These forces encourage build-up rather than breakdown of the bone – increasing its mass and making it stronger. So the more of such exercise you do, the stronger your leg and spinal bones will get in response. Space travel is terrible for bones as there's no gravity acting on them. Astronauts are made to exercise **two and a half hours a day, six days a week** to combat bone loss – and they're usually younger than we are.

Avoiding fractures

It's not surprising we worry about falls as we get older: hip fractures are major injuries, and vertebral fractures cause pain and height loss (see page 132). The evidence is that falls are a bigger risk for fractures than bone weakness on its own. Preventing them is the key to preventing fractures. But bone strength is important too, because IF you fall, you're more likely to fracture a bone if it's weak. We know that stronger muscles correct imbalance more quickly. So if muscle exercises help prevent falls AND strengthen bones, it's clear what we all have to do.

Balance skills themselves are worth practising EVERY DAY – while you brush your teeth for instance. Flip back to the list of things that can make you unsteady (see page 33). Pick up those trip mats and slip mats, watch for side effects of tablets that can cause dizziness or drowsiness (and hence falls), and put your sturdy shoes by the front door in winter, so you don't forget to use them on frosty, wet or icy days.

What you can do for your bones

In both men and women, the bone loss 'gap' can be offset by a healthy balanced diet and plenty of exercise. A good birthday present for a woman aged 59 might be a pair of 3kg weights and a special birthday message: 'Happy 60 Sit-to-Stands, with a 3kg weight in each of your hands' (see page 42).

To keep your bones strong and offset the bone loss 'gap', follow this advice:

- **Increase your activity**: especially the impact type – walking and skipping are good.
- **Increase your strengthening exercises**: these build up muscles but also bone. Stronger muscles reduce your risk of falling. And keep up your balance skills (see page 45–46).
- **Have a healthy, nutritionally balanced diet** containing sufficient calcium (1200 milligrams for a woman, and 1000 milligrams for a man until you're 70, when 1200 milligrams are required). Look at NHS Choices (www.nhs.uk) for examples of calcium-containing foods, e.g. sardines with the bones in (or mackerel or pilchards, mashed and spiced up), soya/tofu, nuts, low fat dairy, broccoli and okra.

- **Ensure you have enough vitamin D** in your diet (oily fish, eggs, fortified spreads and cereals) or by taking simple supplements (see www.nhs.uk for suggestions). Currently, everyone over 65 is recommended to take 10 micrograms) of vitamin D supplement daily. In the summer 10–15 minutes of daily sunlight to face and hands will do.
- **Stop smoking**.
- **Keep your alcohol intake within safe limits**.

HRT is no longer used routinely for bone protection after the menopause as it increases the risk of breast cancer and, sometimes, heart and circulatory problems. New NICE guidelines on managing menopausal symptoms emphasise the importance of a healthy lifestyle, plenty of activity, and sufficient calcium and vitamin D for maintaining bone strength. But it also gives more detail about the risks and benefits of HRT. If, after balancing these, a woman decides HRT is acceptable to control her symptoms, it will help prevent bone thinning too.

Red flags

- **An injured limb**: if you cannot put weight on an injured leg or ankle, you may have broken a bone. **Go to your nearest A&E or dial 999 for an ambulance to take you.**
- **Bone pain at night**: persistent pain deep inside a bone, especially if it wakes you up, needs medical advice.
- **On long-term steroids?** Check you have vitamin D and calcium supplements.

RESOLUTIONS

✓ I will walk as much as possible every day, to strengthen my bones.

✓ If I am a woman I will do 60 sit-to-stands daily, working up gradually to a 3kg weight in each hand.

✓ If I am over 65, I will take a 10 microgram supplement of vitamin D. Otherwise, I will ensure my diet has sufficient vitamin D and calcium.

✓ I will practise my balancing exercises every day.

Take care of your ... Joints

The biomechanics of your joints are super spectacular. Look at the sections on suppleness (page 31) and finding your healthy weight (page 78) – they cover most of what you need to know. Your joints need care, and depend on strong bones and muscles, a 'capsule' keeping lubricating fluid inside and healthy nerve endings to operate smoothly.

Age-related changes

Joint capsules become more fibrous and less resilient, and joints tend to become stiffer more quickly with inactivity, as you get older. The cartilage surfaces become thinner and more fragile. But there is little evidence that age alone, or ordinary activities like walking, cause the commonest problem – osteoarthritis, from which many of us suffer. So what's the explanation?

At the risk of sounding like a broken record, the biggest factor is usually inactivity and weight gain, on top of the cumulative effects of your genetics, other joint diseases (like rheumatoid arthritis, gout or severe joint injuries) and your occupational history. Ballet dancers ruin their toe joints with point work. Footballers damage their knees, because of frequent twisting injuries.

But what tips the balance between manageable problems in weight-bearing joints (which are usually the ones that finally let us down, especially the knees), and more disabling arthritis, is an inactive lifestyle and excess weight. Mechanical joint problems not dealt with by active management (see below) can lead to long-term inactivity and potentially contribute to depression, excess weight, metabolic ill health, type 2 diabetes, further inactivity and more joint disease. It's a downward spiral. But the good news is that you can get off this spiral at any point. You may need to rest an acutely painful joint for a few days, but keep thinking about how to return to activity as soon as safely possible.

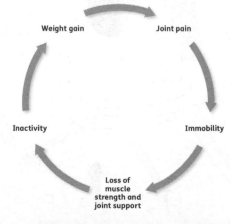

Weight gain   Joint pain

Inactivity   Immobility

Loss of
muscle
strength and
joint support

Fig 5: Basic Cycle of Worsening Joint Pain with
inactivity, weight gain and loss of muscle strength

What you can do for your joints

In general terms, look to your lifestyle to help keep healthy joints. Adopt the following practices:

1. **Your suppleness exercises** (see page 31).
2. **Your core muscle exercises** (see page 39) and WALKING, to maintain your posture and spinal strength.
3. **Special exercises**, if recommended for your joints.
4. **Don't sit too long**, get up and move about to prevent stiffness.
5. **Keep a healthy weight** to avoid overloading your weight-bearing joints.

For minor twists and strains, use First Aid First, then **P**rotect, **R**est, **I**ce, **E**levation, **C**ompression (RICE). After your first aid, a supportive bandage (ask your pharmacist) and anti-inflammatory gels can help. Once the sprained part is adequately rested, gentle mobilising and strengthening exercises that are natural to your joint – like moving up and down on tiptoe when you're getting over a sprained ankle – help rehearse joint-nerve skills, and keep the joint responsive to position change.

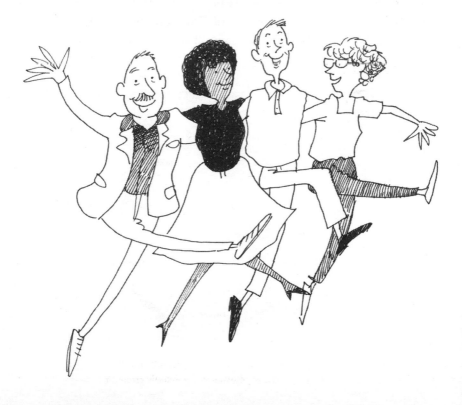

Red flags

Severe, unexplained pain or stiffness in or around one or more joints? Please see your GP.

- **A single hot, red, painful joint** that's exquisitely tender to touch or move is an **emergency** that needs to be sorted the same day. It could be gout (when crystals of uric acid salts are deposited in a joint), or an infected joint potentially needing urgent treatment that day from an orthopaedic specialist.
- **Many joints affected symmetrically**, especially if worse in the morning, may be inflammatory arthritis. You may need referral to a specialist after seeing your GP.

RESOLUTIONS

✓ I will do my **suppleness exercises** (Pearl No. 1, or Chapter 2) every day.

✓ I will do my **strengthening exercises** (Chapter 2) every day.

✓ If I am sitting reading or at work I will set my watch to prompt me to **stretch and flex my joints for two minutes** at least every 20 minutes.

✓ I will **not increase my weight from today**, and take steps to lose excess if I need to (see page 82–86).

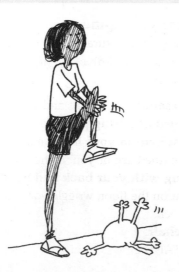

Taking care of your ... Spine

'Walk tall, walk straight and look the world right in the eye'. Whether or not you liked his music, Val Doonican was **the** big TV personality of his day, and is remembered for that very line. It's good advice. So keep it up for as long as possible.

Age-related changes

As you age, there is a tendency to lose your natural spinal curves, lose height (because the intervertebral discs get thinner), and lose spinal bone strength, putting you at risk of fractures if you fall. The problem is that losing your curves makes you less upright, as your head thrusts forwards like a tortoise, and your upper trunk gradually follows suit. This is more unstable, because your centre of gravity is no longer in your plumb line, but in front of it, even more so if you are overweight.

You have three natural spinal curves:

1. Your cervical spine – the neck – curving forwards.
2. Your thoracic spine – the chest – curving backwards.
3. Your lumbar spine – the lower back – curving forwards.

Your neck muscles need to work hard to keep your head up because it's heavy. Similarly, you need to build and maintain your lumbar and core muscles to keep your trunk secure and upright and your lumbar curve intact, so your heavy upper body doesn't pull forward. And walking is good for all these muscles, especially if you maintain your posture.

What you can do for your spine

In addition to protecting your natural spinal curves by building up your posture (see Pearl No. 3, on page 26) and your spinal muscle strength (see page 39), you could also try:

1. **The Alexander technique**, Pilates and T'ai Chi.
2. **Keeping your upright sitting posture** with a box under your feet.
3. **Using a headrest behind your head** and a small cushion behind your lumbar spine (the base of your spine), when driving.
4. **Practise standing with your back and head against the wall**, keep your feet flat on the floor, wriggle your back up the wall, gently stretching your neck.
5. **Beware of the chair**: if you have a desk job, make your desk into a worktop and STAND at it. Standing is the new sitting. Keep your

legs and back muscles strong, your shoulders relaxed not hunched, and your spine erect not crunched or slumped.

6. **Bend it like Beckham, from the knees** – to save your back from unnecessary strain when lifting something from the floor it is much better for your back if you can bend at the knees and then straighten up again, rather than stoop or lean over.

Prevention of vertebral fractures

These can be very painful, restrict mobility and often need strong painkillers until healed. They cause significant loss of height and if a vertebra crushes into a wedge shape they cause angulation of the spine with severe effects on posture. Preventing falls and maintaining bone and muscle strength will help (see pages 32 and 36). It is particularly important to maintain all these preventive steps if you are a woman.

Red flags

- **Persistent pain in your spine** that's still there at night: please see your GP.
- If you have a **family history** or risk factors **for osteoporosis** (see page 125) discuss this with your GP and check you have the necessary vitamin D, calcium and, if recommended, a bone scan to rule out osteoporosis.

RESOLUTIONS

✓ I will keep my head up and face forwards, and my posture plumb line.

✓ I will check that my workstation or laptop is at the right height to stop me hunching over it.

✓ I will increase my walking to build and strengthen my spinal bones and muscles.

✓ I will try to do 5 minutes spinal stretch every day.

✓ I will practice my balance, by standing on one leg, each leg in turn, every day.

Take care of your ... Feet

Your feet are your pivots for walking and your base for standing. They represent millennia of evolutionary changes to keep you upright, even when you're on the move. They are bioengineering masterpieces and deserve the best care you can give them.

Age-related changes

As we age the skin on our feet becomes thinner and less elastic and the myriad of tiny joints in the feet stiffen more quickly with inactivity. However, most age-related changes to the feet are due to decades of **poor footwear, excess weight, inactivity, smoking and the consequences of certain diseases** (not all of which are preventable). High heels and narrow, tight shoes damage feet. They cause internal foot-joint problems, contribute to bunions, corns, calluses and poor posture leading to avoidable extra wear on your knee joints and lumbar spine.

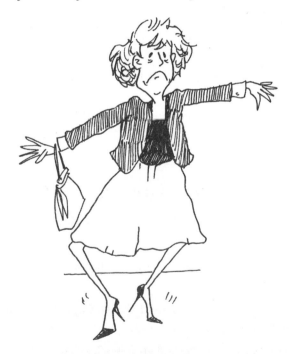

If you have always worn comfy, roomy and well-fitting footwear, and have been lucky to avoid diseases which can damage the joints, skin or nerves of your feet, your feet should continue to serve you well. Ordinary walking and running is not usually associated with damage to the feet and pain and discomfort are not a part of normal age-related change. They always represent other processes at work – sometimes over many years.

Smoking, diabetes and other causes of arterial disease reduce the blood supply to your feet, and diabetes, or other causes of nerve damage, can reduce sensation. This is dangerous because you may not be aware of minor injuries and will be more prone to infections, which quickly become serious. If you are diabetic, sensation and circulation in both your feet should be checked annually.

What you can do for your feet

It's never too late to start looking after your feet. The single most important thing is comfy footwear, with plenty of room for your toes and broad heels to distribute your weight. Good footwear helps your posture and walking, which in turn strengthens your core and leg muscles, keeping you active, upright and independent. Taking care of your tootsies will reap dividends for your health and well-being.

General health and exercise for foot care should include:

- **Exercising your calf muscles**, which move your feet and ankles, and stretch them to avoid the tendons getting tight and the feet stiff (see page 43).
- **Exercising your feet before they hit the floor**: wriggle your toes and rotate your feet and ankles before you get out of bed or up from a chair.
- **Walking**: for muscle strength, strong bones and a healthy circulation.
- **Keep a healthy weight** and take the load off your feet.
- **Stop smoking**, it reduces the circulation to your feet dramatically.
- **Do your heel-to-toe balance exercises** – they help your feet as well as reducing the risk of falls (see page 46).

Red flags

- If you suddenly develop a severely painful white, cold foot even in the warm, especially if you're a smoker or diabetic, please call your GP immediately – it could be a blocked artery.
- If your **feet become numb or tingling**, especially if you're diabetic, see your GP.
- If you develop **ulcers or infections** of your feet or ankles, see your nurse or GP.

- **New or changed moles** on your soles or your toes? See your GP.
- If your **ankles are always swollen** even when it's not hot, see your GP.
- If you have **foot pain that persists and makes walking difficult** check your footwear – discuss with your pharmacist, practice nurse or GP if it persists.

RESOLUTIONS

✓ I will wear shoes that fit and are comfortable.

✓ If I am diabetic or have poor vision I will ask a podiatrist to cut my toenails.

✓ If I am diabetic I will report any ulcers urgently (within 24 hours).

✓ I will treat any infections of my feet before they get worse.

✓ I will thoroughly moisturise my feet every week.

✓ I will do heel raises to strengthen my ankles every day (see page 45).

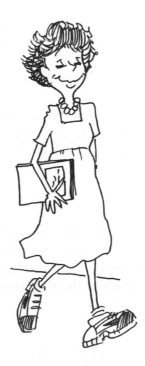

PEARL NO. 9: FINDING YOUR FEET

You need two plastic bowls (big enough to put both feet in, or one at a time), two towels, moisturising cream, one seat:

✓ Fill one bowl with hand-hot water, the other with cool water.

✓ Soak your feet in hand-hot water for 2 minutes, wiggling toes.

✓ Transfer your feet into cool water for 2 minutes, wiggle toes again.

✓ Put your feet back into hand-hot water for 2 more minutes' wiggling.

✓ Dry your feet carefully, especially between the toes.

✓ Rub a grape-size lump of cream into each foot, including between your toes.

✓ Keep rubbing your feet gently until the cream is absorbed.

✓ CAN YOU FIND YOUR FEET? HOW DO THEY FEEL?

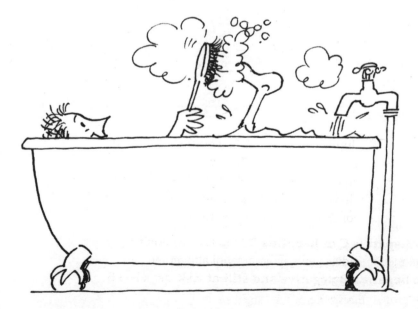

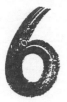

RHYTHM AND BLUES

Sex, drugs (one or two), and rock and roll

First up is your pelvic floor then your sexual health. Then, we'll cover (some more of) your bits: (men's and women's), your waterworks (controlling the flow and troubleshooting the problems) and finally your kidneys.

Take care of your ... Pelvic floor

Whether you're a man or a woman, your pelvic floor is the foundation and muscular framework underpinning your sexual function, and urinary and faecal control.

Your pelvic floor is a thick muscular sling at the very bottom of your body core, on the inside. It supports your pelvic organs, which sit on it, and basically stops them dropping out.

Pelvic floor exercises

Pelvic floor exercises improve your bladder and bowel control. If you're a woman you may remember doing them after childbirth, and now they'll help control minor prolapse of the womb, vagina and bladder and your sex life too (see page 147). But they also help if you're a man too, especially if you've had prostate surgery. Pelvic floor exercises can be do-it-yourself to begin with.

Don't only do these exercises if you have a problem – everyone should do them, because they keep your muscles strong. You'll know if they're helping after about four months of practice. If they're not, then ask your doctor if physiotherapy is appropriate. This is how to identify and then exercise your pelvic floor muscles:

- **Find them first**: when you're having a wee, stop the flow – when you do, you've found them. It's not a good idea to interrupt your urine flow regularly as it may cause flow problems.
- **Empty your bladder before you start your exercises**. Sitting is fine because your tummy and other muscles need to be relaxed, but some people prefer to do these exercises standing up.
- **The routine is one long** (count to 50) **and ten quick** (count to 10) **contractions** (tightening) three times daily. Focus on your pelvic floor muscles and don't worry about anything else. Relax completely between tightening, then tighten up again straight away.

Why not do these exercises whenever you're waiting for the kettle to boil, or next time you're queuing in the supermarket? No one will know.

Take care of your ... Sexual health

Sexual health is part of your fitness and well-being, whatever your level of activity or none, and whatever your sexual orientation. Provided you and your partner are happy, relaxed and willing, unforced, not harmed and not harming, then whatever type and amount of sexual activity you choose and are able to do comfortably is OK. There are some caveats; sex needs to be legal after all. If there are very significant imbalances in your relationship, check out that you are really happy, relaxed and safe. Be true to yourself and with yourself, as this is an important area of your life.

Age-related changes

Changes are not necessarily problems. If you are fit, well and happy with life, your sexual well-being is likely to reflect this. And the reverse is also true. One difference between the genders that sometimes gets overlooked is that men quite commonly continue to father children, whether in the same or a new relationship. Their sperm production, though gradually reducing, continues into extreme old age. So if you are a man, sex will continue to be linked to your reproductive capacity, which is not the case for women. It means that you may still have a need for contraception or, conversely, be concerned about your fertility. Your 50s and 60s are times when your relationships may change – for many different reasons. Safe sex applies now as at any other time.

Mood changes are not an inevitable part of ageing, but sex is a very sensitive indicator of it. **Stress, low mood, lack of sleep, anxiety and depression** are common, and can reduce sexual well-being whether you're a man or a woman. Loss of interest in sex may be a sign of depression, and should be taken seriously. But your 60s could be a time of more personal freedom and greater opportunity to relax, and this can enhance the quality of your sexual life.

What you can do for your sexual health

The most important thing is not to bottle up problems about your sex life. Talk them through with your partner if you can – it's surprising how often people don't. See your GP or sexual health clinic if you have new or ongoing worries, whatever they are.

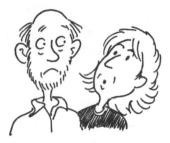

Your sexy six(ty):

1. **Remember the romance and the roses**: the alpha and omega of it all.
2. **Give yourselves time to relax**: remove the pressures and increase the fun.
3. **Lubricate** generously and frequently with a water-based lubricant like KY jelly. Be gentle.
4. **Do your pelvic floor exercises** – start them now! They can help sex, especially if you're a woman.
5. **Your brain is your largest sexual organ**. Use your inventiveness, imagination, playfulness and tenderness. If you're active, have fun with each other – but be safe, always.
6. **You ARE still sexy after surgery, even surgery to your sexy parts**. Give yourself time to adapt, but if your body image is upsetting you, do talk to your partner if you can, and discuss it with your GP. Patience, gentleness, ingenuity and a touch of humour go a long way.

Your Six for Safe(ty):

1. If you're starting a new relationship, **use a condom** (with a water-based lubricant like KY jelly) until you are confident about your sexual health and your partner's.

2. **Impotence CAN be helped – quit smoking**. Impotence (when you can't get an erection) is a red flag to check out your heart, and other issues (see page 142). See your GP. If you're contemplating taking Viagra, or something similar, you need to know it won't work if you are not aroused.
3. **Keep physically and mentally active, and maintain your social life**.
4. **Keep alcohol in safe limits** – it reduces libido (see page 142). In excess it has a negative effect on sexual well-being in men and women.
5. **Lose excess weight** – it helps your pelvic floor.
6. **Stiffness and arthritic change, especially in the hips**. With gentle experimentation, ample uses of pillows and different positions, stiffness and limited movement are usually possible to manoeuvre round. Silk sheets sometimes help.

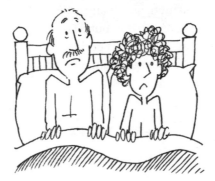

Be confident about your sexual health

Just because you may not need contraception (you won't if you're a woman, but you might if you're a man) doesn't mean you don't need protection. Keep those condoms in your pocket or bag and bring them out in good time.

Sexually transmitted infections (STIs) are increasing in our 60s – the rate has doubled over the last few years in the over 45s. There are more of us singletons about – through divorce, bereavement, or simply single. If you're sexually active … and travelling … you're at risk.

According to NHS Choices (www.nhs.uk) the commonest infections are genital herpes (usually very painful when erupted), genital warts (often visible) and gonorrhoea (which can cause a discharge from your vagina or penis). If these symptoms crop up please get medical advice, either from your GP or, better still, your local sexual health clinic – they're set up to help with as much on-the-spot diagnosis as possible.

But you are at risk of ANY of the STIs if you're unprotected and sexually active, and you're not immune to chlamydia, trichomonas, syphilis, HIV, hepatitis B or C either.

More often than not, STIs happen without you knowing and have no symptoms at all. If you have a sore, ulcer, discharge, or anything unusual about your private parts – please check it out at your local clinic.

Red flags – whether you're a man or a woman

- **Bleeding after sex** – please check this out with your GP.
- **Loss of libido** (loss of interest in your sex life) is NOT part of healthy ageing. If it persists, please see your doctor to rule out physical or mental health problems, or discuss lifestyle factors.
- **Feeling uncomfortable or distressed about any aspect of your sex life.** There may be an emotional, mental or physical problem in your relationship or any aspect of your sexual health. It may flag serious concerns about STIs, or activity forced on you against your wishes. Don't keep problems to yourself – please get help from your GP or sexual health clinic.

RESOLUTIONS

✓ I will remember the romance and the roses. And the occasional poem.

✓ If I have a problem in my sex life I will try to discuss it with my partner if appropriate, but also with my GP or sexual health clinic.

✓ If I have a new partner I will use condoms until infections are excluded.

✓ If I am in a coercive, destructive or violent relationship, I will seek help immediately.

Men matter

This is a sensitive area and it's important to get it right. For men as for women, age-related lifestyle effects, some of which can lead to disease, often swamp healthy ageing.

Age-related changes

Testosterone levels DO drop a bit with age, but if you are healthy, active, don't drink to excess, are not overweight, have not had a head injury or one of the less common diseases that can lead to low testosterone, your levels will only drop a little (certainly not as dramatically as oestrogen levels do in women after their menopause). Your testicles don't stop working. Your sperm and testosterone production continue into very old age, unless lifestyle factors or disease, or both, stop or reduce testicular function.

Healthy age-related changes to your men's bits are likely to be minimal in your 60s. The average length of a man's penis when flaccid is about 3.6 inches, and a little over 5 inches when erect. This changes little with age. In your 60s, the time to ejaculation gradually increases above the average 5.5 minutes (as does the time to a second erection, which may be more difficult to achieve).

If your libido has dropped persistently, it ISN'T just your age. SOMETHING ELSE IS GOING ON, and it needs sorting out. Common causes are stress and depression or, less commonly, low testosterone, typically due to excess alcohol or being overweight. It is a good idea to talk to your GP if you have had testicular surgery, a significant head injury, been on medication to shrink your prostate, or had pituitary gland problems, as all these can reduce testosterone levels.

The take-home point here is that ALCOHOL IS AN IMPORTANT CAUSE OF LOW TESTOSTERONE because it is directly toxic to the testicles **and** causes liver changes leading to increased breakdown of testosterone. So, if you are worried your testosterone level is falling, then improve your lifestyle by reducing alcohol consumption and contact your GP to exclude other causes. It's unlikely you will need testosterone replacement medication, unless you are suffering from a condition that has led to its fall.

Impotence

If you have problems with impotence you are not alone. It affects more than 40 per cent of men aged over 60, and causes great distress. Mechanically, what you need for a good erection is a good blood supply to erectile tissue in the penis and a good switch that can turn it on.

Bearing in mind that good erections normally go hand in hand with libido, the likely causes of a poor switch are stress, low libido, nerve damage (often due to diabetes), and drug side effects (prescribed drugs and alcohol). Poor blood supply to the penis is caused by smoking especially, inactivity, excess weight, raised cholesterol and high blood pressure. Impotence can be the EARLIEST warning of cardiovascular disease in men, even before angina (see page 109).

What you can do to help impotence

The most important thing is not to ignore the problem. Don't be too shy to ask for help. NHS Choices (www.nhs.co.uk) has excellent information on impotence. Many treatments are available in addition to the well-known Viagra, which is not suitable for everyone. Do talk to your partner if you can, but **always see your GP** to discuss the options. And don't be embarrassed; it's a very common problem and GPs understand how difficult it can be for people to talk about it.

Waterworks

By the age of 50, more than 40 per cent of men have problems with their waterworks, and they become even more common in your 60s and beyond. Almost all are due to the enlargement of your prostate gland. This is usually harmless in itself, but urinary problems can erode your self-esteem and affect your sex life.

The pattern of symptoms depends on which parts of your prostate get bigger, and whether the bladder outlet is obstructed and urine gets trapped behind, or whether the bladder itself is irritated and overactive even before it's full, causing an unpleasant sense of urgency to empty it. Collectively, these problems are called **L**ower **U**rinary **T**ract **S**ymptoms, or LUTS for short. Almost any combination of the following clusters can occur:

- **Urine in the bladder trying to get out** ('storage problems'), causing urgency – an uncomfortable and urgent need to pee; sometimes not being able to stop yourself if you can't reach the loo in time – urge incontinence (see page 152); frequency, and getting up at night to pee (*nocturia*).
- **Urine being passed** ('voiding problems'): hesitancy starting, poor stream, intermittent flow with small volumes, dribbling at the end of the stream.
- **Urine being incompletely passed** ('post voiding problems'): with continuing dribbling and a sense of incomplete emptying.

What you can do to help your LUTS

Try to discuss urinary problems with your partner, but the important thing is to see your GP. You should ALWAYS have a rectal examination with new LUTS, to find out whether your prostate gland is enlarged (which it almost certainly will be) but also whether it feels hard or irregular, suggestive of cancer. A prostate (PSA) test may be recommended. But, as is explained in Chapter 8 (see page 201), a raised PSA result doesn't mean a diagnosis of prostate cancer, and further investigation is needed.

MILK YOUR URETHRA

Sometimes the urethra itself develops little reservoirs of urine inside it, causing dribbling after your main flow. Try 'milking' your urethra. With gentle pressure, move your thumb or finger along the length of your penis underneath, starting from the back. Bring your finger firmly forwards along the shaft, and repeat this several times. Hopefully, you will 'milk' the residual urine trapped in your urethra, and prevent those wet patches that sometimes appear on your trousers.

Age-related changes

An **inguinal hernia** is a weakness in the muscles of your lower abdominal wall that the contents behind can bulge through. The following can help prevent hernia developing or increasing in size:

- Prevent and treat constipation (see page 119).
- Build up your core abdominal muscles (see page 39).
- Lift things carefully.
- Reduce coughing; give up smoking.

If you're **on medication** (common in your 60s), please discuss any side effects with your pharmacist or GP, especially if you think they are affecting you libido or potency. If excess weight is hiding your penis, losing weight will help restore it to its normal length.

Cancers specific to men

Prostate cancer

There are nearly 40,000 new cases of prostate cancer diagnosed each year. It is the most common cancer in men, and the second commonest cause of death from cancer in men. More research is needed, because we really don't know why this is. The *good* news is that the 10-year survival rate is about 84 per cent. There is no good evidence that ordinary prostate enlargement leads to prostate cancer. But because harmless (benign) enlargement is so common, it is inevitable that some men will develop prostate cancer who did have harmless enlargement before.

Other cancers

Cancer of the testicles is relatively rare in your 60s and beyond, but occasionally develops. If you think your testicle feels odd or hard, or lumpy, please check it out with your GP, ASAP. The success rate of treatment is excellent.

Cancer of the penis (penile cancer) is also rare, but more common after the age of 60. This risk is increased with smoking, but also with genital warts, caused by the human papilloma virus. If you develop any sores, skin changes, or unpleasant penile discharge, please see your GP.

Red flags

The message with any worrying problems affecting your sexual or urinary health, or any aspect of your genitalia is: IF IN DOUBT – CHECK IT OUT!

- **Blood in your urine – please, ALWAYS check this out.**
- **Urinary (waterworks) symptoms (LUTS) –** need checking with your GP. At the same time you should have your prostate examined to assess size and exclude prostate cancer (see page 155).
- **Problems with your penis** – whether or not you are sexually active, if you develop sores, discharge, or anything else that worries you, see your GP or sexual health clinic.
- **Swellings in your scrotum or near your testicles** – most will be harmless cysts of your sperm ducts or hernia, but sometimes they are more serious, or early changes of cancer. Swellings need checking – please see your GP.
- **If you have a family history of prostate cancer,** please discuss this with your GP.

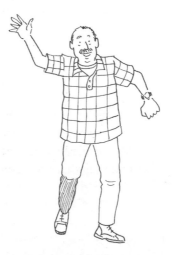

> ## RESOLUTIONS
>
> ✓ If I have urinary problems I will talk to my GP about them, and ask for help.
>
> ✓ I will discuss any erectile dysfunction with my GP.
>
> ✓ I will use condoms in a new relationship until our sexual health is checked.
>
> ✓ I will report blood in my urine.
>
> ✓ I will check out unexplained swellings, ulcers, or worries about my sexual health, promptly.

Women matter

Life is often better after the menopause, on average at about 52 in Western society. Hot flushes have usually settled unless you've just stopped HRT. You've finished with cyclical breast pain and heavy, painful periods. You've said goodbye to PMT forever and put menopausal sleep problems to bed. Hurrah! However, the considerable silver linings (and even 50 shades of grey) don't always compensate for the downside of lower oestrogen. Likely changes you will notice include vaginal dryness, urinary problems, loss of pelvic floor muscle tone, dryness and itchy perineum and a downturn in your body image. However, don't despair, help is on the way.

There is much you can do: increasing your activity and exercise level (See Chapters 2 and 5), practising your pelvic floor exercises (see page 137), using ample lubrication and considering intra-vaginal oestrogen (see page 147) are all helpful. HRT for the whole body ('systemic' HRT) counteracts post-menopausal changes and the temporary hot flushes, sleep and mood disturbances. But it has been used much less for several years, due to concerns about increased risk of breast cancer and heart and circulatory diseases. The National Institute for Clinical Excellence and Health (NICE, www.nice.org.uk) has published new guidelines for managing the menopause. These are based on detailed analysis of the benefits and harms of different types of HRT started in one's 50s (nearer the menopause) rather than in your 60s. But if you have problems, or started HRT in your 50s and are still on it, these guidelines will help discussions with your GP, or prompt referral to a menopause specialist. For some women, the balance of benefit and harms may be acceptable.

PROLAPSE: DOWN BELOW YOUR PELVIC FLOOR

If you're a woman, the drop in oestrogen after your menopause reduces the strength of your pelvic floor muscles, adding to any weakness from overstretch and damage during vaginal childbirth. This contributes to prolapse, (and stress incontinence). The vaginal walls become less elastic too.

✓ **Womb prolapse**. If your pelvic floor muscles cannot support your womb it sags lower into your vagina, causing a dragging sensation.

✓ **Vaginal wall prolapse.** Your vaginal walls can sag towards the vaginal entrance too. The front wall can drag the lower part of the bladder with it, making a bulge into the vagina (*cystocele*). This contributes to dribbling after you think you've emptied your bladder. Sagging of the back wall causes the rectum to bulge in (*rectocele*).

✓ **Sex, and your perception of prolapse**. The evidence is that it's less the amount of prolapse but more how bad you THINK it is that causes problems. This means that surgery for prolapse doesn't always help sex – a recent study showed that one in three woman with prolapse had much improved sexual function after a few months of regular pelvic floor exercises: a great example of an alternative to surgery that can work very well.

What you can do to offset post-menopausal issues:

- **Lubrication for vaginal dryness**. Lubricate generously and frequently with a water-based lubricant (KY jelly or a longer lasting alternative – ask your pharmacist), it helps prevent soreness and reduce friction during intercourse, which can inflame your urethra, making cystitis more likely.
- **Intra-vaginal oestrogen**: as creams or pessaries (tablets which melt inside the vagina) improves natural lubrication, elasticity and comfort. You don't have to be sexually active to use it – it reduces the risk of repeated cystitis anyway. It is essential to use intra-vaginal oestrogen before your cervical smear. Intra-vaginal oestrogen also works well with your pelvic floor exercises to prevent, or improve, stress incontinence. Worth discussing with your GP.

- **Manage your urinary symptoms and continence problems** (see page 151). Remember: always wipe from front to back to reduce the risk of cystitis, and if you think you have cystitis (a burning sensation when you wee and feeling you need to go all the time), drink plenty of fluids straightaway. If the symptoms don't settle in a day or two, please see your pharmacist or GP, as you may need antibiotics. Urinary frequency that persists, or ANY suggestion of blood in your urine, should always be reported.
- **Pelvic floor exercises** (see page 137–138) can help your sex life and improve stress incontinence, prolapse and wind control (see page 117). And avoid straining – (see page 119 for a reminder of how to 'get things moving').
- **Reducing vulval and perineal itch**. Avoid nylon tights and wear cotton pants. Moisturise your perineum (E45 or aqueous cream can help). Consider thrush – ask your pharmacist if an anti-fungal cream or pessary would help. If itching persists, please see your GP for an examination (with a urine sample to check for infection or clues to diabetes) – don't just discuss it. Occasionally a referral to a vulval clinic is needed.
- **Check your perineum for new moles**, and sore spots – you'll need to use a mirror. **And don't forget cycling and saddle sores**. Get a comfy saddle, and check you're not getting sore if you use an exercise bike.
- **Keep a healthy weight and maintain your muscles**: keep active and do your body core and hip exercises. Remember walking and T'ai Chi.
- If your pelvic floor exercises, with or without vaginal oestrogen, haven't managed to control your **stress incontinence** (see page 152) or your prolapse or sexual comfort, you may want to discuss alternative approaches, including surgery, with your GP.

Looking after your breasts

Your main concern is to watch out for changes suggesting possible breast cancer – lumps in your breasts or armpits, discharge from your nipples or skin changes around them (soreness, scaliness like eczema, persistent itch and roughness) or on the breasts themselves.

It is important that you pick up on anything unusual as soon as possible. Pay attention to your breasts whenever you wash or put on moisturiser, and feel them attentively with the flat of both hands all the way to your armpits – so you pick up subtle changes more readily. Look at the appearance of the skin – is it swollen, puckered or odd in any way? If you are concerned about anything that may be flagging up cancer, check it out ASAP.

There may be a simple explanation, for example lymph glands in your armpits fighting off infection from a recent arm-shave. But, **if in doubt check it out**. And don't forget simple things to keep your breasts comfortable. We may be the 'ban the bra' generation, but a bit more support when jogging, and a little TLC, is great, so:

- Wear a good supportive bra, with wide straps, when jogging or exercising.
- Keep up your plumb-line posture.
- Moisturise the skin well.
- Dry carefully under your breasts, and if the skin is itchy or sore ask your pharmacist if an antifungal cream might help, and see your GP if it doesn't.

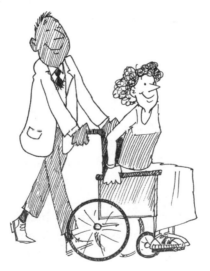

Breast cancer

This is the commonest cancer in the UK and the commonest in women (nearly 50,000 new cases each year). The overall lifetime risk for women is 1 in 8, but more than three-quarters (80 per cent) of breast cancer is in women over 50 years of age, rising higher in women from 65–69 years of age. So it's common among female baby boomers.

Your individual risk of breast cancer in your 60s is less likely to be due to a genetic risk than in women under the age of 50, in whom the BRCA1 and 2 genes (BReast CAncer) are more often involved. Having had children (or any pregnancies) and breastfeeding, reduces your risk. Use of the oral contraceptive pill or HRT increases it. But five years after stopping HRT your risk is no longer affected by it, and remember – **intra-vaginal oestrogen doesn't increase your risk**. You can't change your genetics or your past: so concentrate on what you *can* do. Find your healthy weight and keep alcohol in safe limits, as excess weight and alcohol both increase breast cancer risk.

Unwelcome though a diagnosis of breast cancer is, the good news is that over three-quarters of women (78 per cent) survive at least 10 years after their diagnosis and treatment. See Susie's Solution (page 197) for an example of negotiating difficult decisions about treatment.

Breast screening

Breast Screening is a **backup** for early breast cancer you may not feel, but **always report a breast lump** or any changes suggesting cancer. NHS breast screening in women is currently every three years from 50 to 70, but pilot areas are extending the range to 47–73. You have to make the decision to accept or opt out, as you will be routinely invited unless you have made clear you do not want to be. For more information about breast cancer, and cancer of the womb (the fourth commonest female cancer), the ovaries (the fifth commonest), the cervix (about 2 per cent of female cancers, or just over 3000 new cases each year, and getting more common in our late 60s – after cervical screening has stopped), and the vulva (quite rare) please see www.nhs.uk and www.cancerresearchuk.org.

Red flags

If you are worried about any aspect of your sexual health, genital tract or waterworks, please see your GP. **And report any of the following PROMPTLY to exclude early signs of cancer**:

- **Breast changes**: lumps, nipple changes, persistent unusual discomfort in your breast, or changes to the skin (see above).
- **Vaginal bleeding** after your menopause (postmenopausal bleeding), including bleeding after intercourse (post coital bleeding). Occasionally it's due to cancer of the womb or cervix.
- **New, persistent urinary problems** (including persistent frequency) can occasionally be a warning of bladder cancer, or ovarian cancer which can press on the bladder.
- **Blood in your urine**, even just the once. Occasionally, it is due to bladder cancer, or cancer of the womb or cervix.

- **New and persistent lower abdominal swelling and fullness** is occasionally due to cancer of the ovary – if it's new to you in your 60s, please **don't** assume it's just irritable bowel syndrome.
- **Persistent itch of your vulva** (the lips) that doesn't respond to simple moisturisers or antifungal treatment, or other persistent vulval skin changes **(including moles).**

More often than not, there will be simple explanations for these problems: but they are **ALWAYS** red flags to check out with your GP.

RESOLUTIONS

✓ I will do my pelvic floor exercises every day.

✓ I will use plenty of lubrication during sex.

✓ I will report **any breast lumps** promptly.

✓ I will report **blood** in my urine, on my pants or after intercourse.

✓ I will report **urinary symptoms** promptly to my GP.

Continence: controlling your flow

This is about keeping control of your urine flow: or regaining it if it's gone. You want control, hard won as a toddler. We're talking about embarrassing leaks, ridiculously urgent calls, and sometimes flooding. They're major obstacles to planning your day. You may even have stopped going out for fear you might not find a loo. That is a desperate state and needs help as soon as possible.

Age UK reported that about 3.2 million people age 65 and over suffer from urinary incontinence, with about one in three women and one in seven men affected: so twice as common in women. **START YOUR PELVIC FLOOR EXERCISES NOW!**

And as we will see in Chapter 8, just because you have a problem doesn't mean you need medical treatment. But continence problems can ruin your quality of life; so you need a clear plan. And, if you opt for self-help first (see below) after discussing it with your GP first, have a clear idea about what the next steps will be if your efforts don't work. And sometimes you DO need treatment straight away, to make life bearable.

If you're a man, problems are likely to be LUTS, due to your prostate getting bigger (see Men Matter page 141). If you're a woman, your waterworks problems are usually the result of your weakened pelvic floor muscles, resulting from your childbirth history and the effects of post-menopausal low oestrogen. NHS Choices (www.nhs.uk) is an excellent resource for advice on this.

Incontinence

Stress incontinence is the commonest, mainly affecting women, but it can happen in men, occasionally after prostate surgery. It causes small to medium leaks you may be unaware of – until you spot wet patches on pants or trousers. Coughing, sneezing, laughing, running jumping or straining puts extra pressure on the bladder and can overcome weakened pelvic floor and urethral muscles, making you spring a leak.

Urgency is uncomfortable and you know about it. It's an abnormal need to pass urine before the bladder is full, due to irritation and over-activity of the bladder muscles. When it cannot be controlled, the bladder automatically empties its contents, causing **urge incontinence**. It is the most common type of incontinence in men, usually due to prostate enlargement, but common in women too in whom it can co-exist with stress incontinence.

If you have waterworks problems it is ESSENTIAL to see your GP if you haven't yet, so please do and take a fresh, midstream urine sample with you (see page 158–159) in order to diagnose the problem and its cause as well as excluding any underlying conditions.

WHEN YOU HAVE WATERWORKS PROBLEMS, YOUR GP NEEDS TO EXCLUDE:

✓ **Urine infection**.

✓ **Prostatitis in men** – uncomfortable inflammation, sometimes with infection, of the prostate.

✓ **Diabetes** (a clue is glucose in your urine) – causing increased frequency.

✓ **Prostate cancer** – men with LUTS usually have simple prostate enlargement but, with new symptoms, your GP needs to examine your prostate to rule out signs of cancer.

✓ **Gynaecological cancers** in women – persistent frequency or blood in the urine.

✓ **Bladder cancer** – blood in the urine, sometimes urinary frequency.

✓ **Bladder stones** – minerals in the urine occasionally form lumps in the bladder causing pain. They are commoner in men because prostate enlargement can stop the bladder from emptying completely, so deposits build up.

✓ **Medication side effects**.

Don't forget that STIs can also cause urinary problems, so mention these if it's a possibility. Your GP may recommend further tests, but discuss whether it's reasonable to start the following self-help for continence problems.

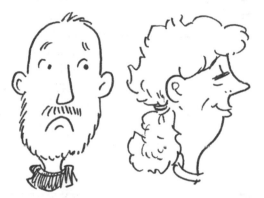

What you can do to help incontinence

There is a lot you can do, whether you're a man or a woman. Here is some general advice, but if progress is an uphill struggle, go back to your GP to discuss drugs (which can be life-transforming), and even surgery:

- **Get more active physically and mentally** – keep your brain alert for continence control.
- **Restrict your fluid intake after 6–7pm** to avoid getting up at night for a wee.
- **Keep alcohol within safe limits** – it irritates the bladder and is a diuretic (like caffeine-containing drinks), making you pass more urine.
- **Manage stress incontinence**: by doing pelvic floor exercise (see page 137), consider intra-vaginal oestrogens (if you're a woman) and deal with your lifestyle.

- **Manage urge incontinence** with bladder retraining (see below) and reducing bladder irritants like caffeine, red squash, alcohol and smoking.

Bladder retraining: managing the urgent urge

Bladder retraining uses your brainpower, nerve power and the power of your pelvic floor and urethral tightening muscles (under your control) to get **you** in control of your urge, rather than your irritated (and irritating) bladder.

Retraining works by gradually increasing the intervals between emptying your bladder, so it learns to fill up a bit more before urging you to relieve yourself.

If you cannot control urgency, your bladder will empty its full contents.

You need a day to plan how to build your bladder tolerance, logging every time you go for a pee. Work out the average interval between visits to the loo. If you went eight times, with seven intervals of 100, 45, 100, 60, 45, 30, 60 minutes, the average interval would be 63 minutes. Then work out your target interval, which is your average interval plus 15 minutes (so in our example, the target interval would be 78 minutes).

- On **Day One** of your retraining, aim to hold on to your urine for the target interval after emptying your bladder. If you think you cannot make it, tighten up hard, as best you can, and slowly walk to the loo. You mainly use your pelvic floor muscles to do this, so your exercises are ESSENTIAL.
- If you need to work up to your target interval more gradually, remember you **must** wait a bit longer than your old average interval.
- Keep going, it will take a few weeks to notice the benefit so plan to review things with your GP when you have tried for 4–6 weeks.

Toilet tips for men and women

If you dribble after you you've finished:

- **Spend two pennies**. After the first, wait a minute, and go again.
- **If you're a man: urine may be pooling in your urethra**. Try 'milking' your urethra (see page 144).
- **If you're a woman: it may be due to a small cystocele** (see page 147). After emptying your main flow, try standing up, it may help drain your dribble.

Other issues:

- **If you're a man: hesitancy and slow stream at the start** will be your prostate getting in the way. Try sitting down on the loo, it may help urine flow by slightly increasing the pressure on your bladder.
- **Always wash your hands after visiting the loo** – especially if you've done a helpful manoeuvre.

Emergency supplies

Pads, liners and disposable pants for men and women are available from pharmacies and most large supermarkets. Many people in their 60s (and before) have a spare pair of pants (or two), tucked somewhere for the occasional accident. Change wet pants ASAP, to stop the skin getting sore, and to reduce odour.

If you're struggling, you can apply to the NKS (link at NHS Choices) for a RADAR key, to use toilets for the disabled. The Bladder and Bowel Foundation (phone 01536 533 255) or online (info@bladderandbowelfoundation. org) can provide you with a nationally recognised card, entitling you to use the convenience if challenged.

Other solutions

If your efforts to sort out problems with your waterworks have not worked, you need to review the next steps with your GP. Specialist physiotherapy may help finesse pelvic floor exercises. There are many drugs and sometimes surgery to help. Having tried without first, you'll have a better idea how essential they might be. You always need to discuss possible side effects of medication with your GP, especially if you're on other drugs as well.

THE WATERWORKS MEDICINE BOX

Discuss the possibilities with your GP. Drugs can help:

✓ **Urgency and urge incontinence** in both sexes. They reduce bladder irritability. Avoid drugs detrimental to brain function (if used for long enough at high doses). There are several to choose from.

✓ **Obstruction to urine outflow.** Drugs can relax muscles around the bladder neck (not under conscious control). They may lower blood pressure.

✓ **Shrink the prostate in men**, when LUTS are troublesome. The common one is finasteride. It reduces testosterone levels so can have side effects, reducing libido. They need to be taken long-term to shrink the prostate.

✓ **Urethral irritation and recurrent cystitis in women:** intra-vaginal oestrogen (see page 147).

✓ **Stress incontinence in women**: very occasionally drugs, as well as local oestrogen and pelvic floor exercises, are used.

If LUTS, or stress incontinence, has not responded to self-help, exercises or drugs then surgery may need considering.

Surgery to remove the prostate in men (prostatectomy) is much better than it was and is usually done via the urethra (through the penis). This makes it much safer. Older forms of surgery occasionally cause stress incontinence. If you've had prostate surgery (and even if not), please take care when you cycle: ensure your saddle is comfy and not rubbing the skin.

Surgery for stress incontinence in women can be helpful and there are many approaches. They all have potential side effects and are not always successful, but can be extremely effective when all else has failed!

Red flags

The following symptoms require immediate attention from your GP:

- **Bleeding when you pass urine** ALWAYS needs an explanation. It is often simple infection, but occasionally due to bladder cancer, or cancer of the lining of the womb in women, and further tests will be advised.
- **Waves of severe pain on passing urine** – at the tip of the urethra, your lower tummy or back may be due to a stone.
- **In women, new but persistent frequency,** especially if it's associated with a sense of fullness in your lower tummy, may be an ovarian cyst or cancer.

RESOLUTIONS

✓ I will drink sufficient water daily, but restrict fluids after 7pm.

✓ I will report bleeding in my urine straight away.

✓ I will report new waterworks symptoms to my GP.

✓ I will do my pelvic floor exercises.

The source of the flow: care of your kidneys

Your waterworks begin with your kidneys, tucked inside you in your lumbar region.

Your kidneys extract waste material from your blood, preventing toxicity. Together with your large bowel they control your body's overall water balance. Humans can live for about three weeks without food, but cannot survive for more than a few minutes without oxygen, or a few days without water.

So the most important thing you can do for your waterworks is to drink sufficient water (at least 6–8 full glasses of fluid daily). When you do it is another matter, and restricting it after 7pm helps reduce the number of times you get up at night to pee.

Age-related changes

Kidney function declines a little with age, but in the absence of disease this will not affect your health or well-being. As with **all those other bits of you** that need looking after as you get older, so too your kidneys are affected by your level of fitness and its affect on their blood supply. Many common diseases and conditions including high blood pressure and type 2 diabetes are related to your lifestyle. They can contribute to how well your kidneys work, as can a history of infection, kidney stones and other conditions, your family and occupational history, and your medication.

What you can do to help your kidneys

The most important things you can do to take care of your kidneys are:

- **Drink sufficient water** – at least 6–8 full glasses a day – but more in hot weather or as you do more exercise. This helps prevent kidney stones that can develop when the urine becomes too concentrated.

- **Keep up your fluid intake when you are ill**, especially with diarrhoea, vomiting or fever. High fevers make you sweat more so you lose water, and if you're being sick or have diarrhoea you're losing fluids too.
- **Keep active and keep a healthy weight**.
- **Stop smoking**.
- **Keep your alcohol in safe limits**.
- **Keep a watery eye on your medication**, is it affecting your urine output?
- **If you have severe, acute diarrhoea, please ask** your doctor whether you should stop any medication temporarily.

Red flags

- At the risk of sounding like a record stuck in a groove, **always check out blood in your wee**.
- **Report any fever associated with pain in your kidneys** (either side of your lumbar region), especially with other symptoms like a burning feeling when you wee. It could be serious kidney infection needing urgent medical assessment.
- **Report waves of severe pain in your kidneys**, the lower side of your tummy, above your pubic bone and (if you are a man) the tip of your penis, that come on when you want to pee. They could be due to a stone (formed from minerals in your urine if it's too concentrated). Stones can get stuck somewhere along your urinary tract, causing one of the worst pains there is. It needs urgent medical assessment.
- **If you cannot pass urine**, the first thing is to try to relax, keep warm, and see if that helps. But if you can't, it is essential to seek medical advice promptly.
- **If your urine flow is decreasing** noticeably day by day, for no obvious reason (such as not drinking enough fluids), please seek medical advice.

KIDNEY PROBLEMS NEED A URINE SAMPLE

If you have a problem that may be to do with your kidneys, please see you doctor AS SOON AS POSSIBLE and take a **fresh urine sample** with you. The best thing to do is to arrive a bit early for your appointment, ask the receptionist for a sample bottle, and pass a MID-STREAM SAMPLE in to it. That means go to the loo with your bottle and uncap it. Then with your bottle in one hand, let the first dribbles of urine pass into the pan (washing away debris, from your urethra or crotch, which might affect the sample) and then catch your sample from the next bit of flow – fresh from the bladder. Just a little will do. Replace the cap and screw it tight shut.

If you know you will find this contortion difficult, ask the receptionist if there is a nurse or health care assistant who can help you.

RESOLUTIONS

✓ I will keep up my daily fluid intake: about one and a half litres, or 6–8 glasses (including my unsweetened tea, coffee or soft drinks), and increase how much I drink in hot sweaty weather.

✓ I will keep active, keep a healthy weight, stop smoking and keep my blood pressure under control.

✓ If I have blood in my urine I will report this to my doctor promptly.

STUFF HAPPENS

The good, the bad and the ugly

There are many life-enhancing events to look forward to in your 60s, whether you retire, change directions or extend your existing career. You may finally have the chance to pick up both old and new interests. You could build a garden wall, go hiking, write a book, visit far-flung relatives, learn a new language, volunteer or campaign for social and political change. There may be the anticipation – or arrival – of grandchildren, grand nieces and nephews, and a sense of many futures ahead.

A recent report showed that there was a reduction of 25 per cent in the number of visits retirees made to their GP, compared with non-retirees. The explanation seems to be: less stress, more good quality sleep at night, and more exercise and physical activity.

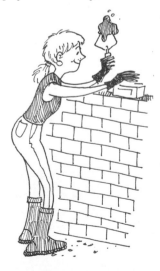

In this chapter, we'll also look at some life events that can be tough to handle: being a carer, bereavement, divorce and facing one's own death, which we will all have to do one day. But the stuff of everyday life can hit hard too: falling out with a friend, financial worries, or things not going well at work. Stuff can creep up on us as we find we've got more and more commitments and demands on our time. When we don't know which way to turn, something's going to go pop if we don't do something about it.

While we all react in different ways when the shit hits the fan, the important thing to remember is not that 'stuff happens', because we know it will, it's how we react to it that counts. We can't predict everything and we don't really know how we'll feel when whatever happens actually happens; but we can prepare for it and decide NOW that we'll manage the stuff as best we can.

Facing a build-up of ordinary things, major transitions or unwanted life events can cause stress, poor sleep, low mood, panic attacks and anxiety. If unsupported and unmanaged, these can escalate into emergencies: suicidal thoughts, dangerous behaviour putting you and others at risk, or unwise decisions that have consequences that are difficult to reverse. These are red flags that say: 'I'm not waving, I'm drowning'. If you don't have good coping strategies you'll be more likely to use bad ones: increased drinking, smoking, comfort eating and withdrawal, leading to isolation, loss of confidence and self-esteem and possibly worse. So, let's decide now that it's worth coping as best you can at the outset.

Don't give up

Many of us in our 60s will remember the Scout motto: 'Be Prepared', which referred to preparedness of body and mind to do the right thing at the right time. What really matters here is not how perfect preparation is, but whether it helps. Every bit of help in life is worth it, whatever the appearance to the contrary. Don't give up trying to move in the direction you want to go, unless you feel you're on the wrong path. In which case, get off it as quickly as is safely possible.

We're about to think of some of the major challenges: those that hit us like a tsunami, and those that build up relentlessly over time, and can overpower us. Our preparations should be based on three things: firstly fostering a resilient attitude, secondly, gathering the resources that we need to help us (and others) and, thirdly, taking on board the reality of what has happened. One of the key resources we need is mindfulness (see page 62), as this will help us live in the present, learn from the past and plan for the future.

Facing stuff when it happens

This is not just about adapting to stress and adversity, but coping constructively with it so it doesn't overpower and defeat you. Building resilience and being prepared starts long before stuff happens. The whole point of coping as best one can is to come out the other side, and help others to do so too. Consider the following tools that you can use to help face the Bad and the Ugly.

Resources and resilience

Don't forget your own resilience and resources, gathered, grown and developed throughout your life. This is the first strength you call upon, and it will be there for you. You have 60 years of living under your belt, and you didn't get here without picking up a few tricks along the way. Don't panic, try the Long Goodbye to control it (see Pearl No: 10, on page 171).

You can learn from your own past. In difficult and challenging times, what were your strengths and what was hard? How did you manage? What, if any, are the pitfalls you'd want to avoid this time? You don't need to wait for stuff to happen to answer these questions, better to do it when you're not too preoccupied to look. Everything that builds your physical, mental, emotional and social well-being contributes to your resilience.

Preparedness

There is much you can do to prepare strong foundations to support you during life's more unwanted events. We make plans in advance for lesser things in our life, so why not the bigger things too? Here's a brief checklist of things you might want to consider doing:

- Your will.
- Advanced decisions about your health and well-being (see Chapter 8).
- A flag to the location of a key document or the contact details of a trusted person who knows where it is kept.
- A clear list of your key contacts (in case you lose your mobile).
- A list of what is essential to have to hand when or if stuff happens.

But you know you. You may not like to think too much about the future, and prefer to meet most things, however difficult, if or when they come. That's OK. But remember that you may need more time to orientate yourself when stuff happens. Take time to work out exactly what is going on when you do face challenging stuff, so you can bring your own resources to it, as well as seek any other help you need. This preparedness is likely to help you feel more in control.

A good place to start your preparations is the internet, as there is much helpful advice. Trusted sites are worth starting with (see page 203), and you won't go far wrong if you start with NHS Choices (www.nhs.uk), where the combined knowledge and experience of hundreds of health professionals, therapists and advisors has been drawn together. It is an impressive resource, regularly updated.

Experiencing and facing the reality

Even when major life events hit hard, you can limit the damages. You can try to get things under control and stabilised, and then shrink the damage as best you can, so that your own life, and the lives of others too, are not derailed. But as we all know: some stuff can be **very** bad, **very** ugly and potentially **very** damaging. You may feel, temporarily, as if life has been shaken to its core.

Remember your holistic route to well-being (see page 54). Guard your sleep, eat regular meals of Mediterranean food. Keep up your 10-minute Triple S routine (it's essential). Practice mindful breathing, and bring your mindful gaze to the present. Keep in touch with friends and family. Be true to yourself **and** with yourself (see page 54) and watch out for harms.

Important as it is to be able to comfort others, you also need to take care of your own reactions, knowing the person you are. Remember the advice about oxygen masks when you fly? Put yours on first, *then* help someone else. This is part of being true to yourself and with yourself. Being true **to** yourself means that you too, like others, will have your own way of reacting and dealing with things – hopefully strengthened by the resilience you have built and the resources you can access when you need. Being true **with** yourself means keeping a watchful, caring eye **on** yourself too. Are things really OK? Do you need help? Are things really just too much to bear? Do you need something or someone to help support you, even if only temporarily?

Our reactions to life's tougher events inevitably bring out our individual as well as our common needs. There is no single way of reacting to stuff that happens in life, but the following characteristics, not in any strictly fixed order, usually ring true. You will probably recognise these features if you have previously experienced a major loss or an unwanted event.

They are discussed on the NHS Choices website for bereavement (a good resource), but they have more general applications too:

- **accepting** the reality
- **experiencing** the pain
- **adjusting** to your loss
- **putting less energy into grieving** (for whosoever or whatever it is that is lost).

Coping with stuff

On a choppy sea you need good gear: a first aid kit, a lifebelt and maybe a life raft. If there's a red flag waving, it's good to know there's a lifeline connecting you to the shore, and an even greater reassurance that there's a lifeboat you can call if needed, to take you to safety.

Rehearsal, hands on or imaginative, **is part of the preparation** for an emergency. Reading helpful advice flags it up, but what really matters is whether you can use it at the right time. Health care professionals have to rehearse their resuscitation skills, even if they only use them a few times.

You need some **portable lifebelts.** The following three are worth practising in advance, so they are second nature whenever you need them:

- Positive Reflections at Bedtime (Pearl No. 7, see page 65).
- The Long Goodbye (Pearl No. 10, see page 171).
- Deep, Deep Relaxation (Pearl No. 11, see page 187).

It boosts well-being to look for good things. This doesn't put a rosy gloss on life, but counters the tendency to ignore the good when overwhelmed by the bad and ugly – including your own negative thoughts.

There are some other portable lifebelts you can prepare in advance:

A real first aid kit! Be practical – have a real one for your bathroom cabinet and your car, and a few sticking plasters in your wallet or purse. Consider:

- **An emergency overnight bag**: with the basics – a spare toothbrush, night clothes, pants and socks – just in case. Shove it in a cupboard till you need it.
- **A personal survival bag**: with a few things inside that really matter to you: a photograph or two of those you love, a good book, or even a small tool kit if you can't bear to be without a screwdriver.

- **A list of important and emergency contact numbers**, with a copy in your home for others to see if they need to – stick it on the fridge or next to the land line, and give a copy to a good friend. Put a copy in your overnight bag too.
- **Copies of key documents collected in a file** (and online) – advanced plans you might have, or practical personal details. Flag up the location of these, for emergencies.

Always remember, you are not alone. There are lots of people who can help you, some of whom are so obvious we sometimes forget them when caught up in stuff.

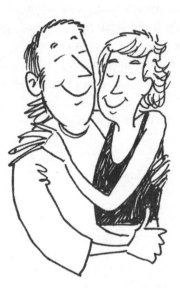

YOUR LIFE RAFTS, LIFELINES AND LIFEBOATS

✓ Friends and family.

✓ Your GP, pharmacist, specialist or District Nurse.

✓ The Samaritans (telephone: 116-123; email: jo@samaritans.org).

✓ Your work colleagues, work counselling, your Trade Union.

✓ Alcoholics Anonymous (0800-9177-650, alcoholics-anonymous. org.uk).

✓ Citizens Advice Bureau (CAB).

✓ Your local priest, minister, rabbi, imam or Elder.

✓ Your lawyer.

✓ Your list of important contacts.

Common red flags: the five big Ds

Things can happen when you haven't got the resilience or the resources to cope with stuff. It's important to prevent them if you can, but just as important to get help if they happen. It's not a sign of weakness to realise you need help; it's the first step in solving the problem and halfway to coming out the other side. So never hold back from getting the help you need.

Watch out for:

- Depression
- Despair
- Drink
- Drugs (prescription mainly)
- Debt

Moving on

Moving on is less about getting over something, and more about incorporating the reality of it into the rest of your life. It is not pretending that a crisis, loss or life event hasn't happened, but recognising it is no longer centre stage all the time. You can attend to other aspects of your life, and the lives of others too.

Some stressful scenarios

However painful many of these are, coping with them can reveal unexpected opportunities for personal growth. Even facing death may bring reconciliation and peace that one never dreamt of. So the toughest times, though never sought, may have hidden boons.

The squeezed middle

Life has events – but they're not always the problem. It may be a state of 'being' where everybody needs you all the time. If it continues for days, weeks and months – without an end in sight – it can be overwhelming. It can sap your energy, lower your mood and make you feel that you've lost touch with yourself. If you have, you may have lost touch with other people too, even though you're with them most of the time. This is called stress, in one of its many guises. And if it's making you panic: try Pearl No. 10: The Long Goodbye, on page 171.

If you're in a squeezed middle, caring for grandchildren or your own children for example, helping aged parents, and struggling with your own life stresses as well – you're pulled in all directions. You're balancing X, Y and Z, juggling a lot of balls – dropping a few – swivelling round to catch them and at risk of falling over.

But you are not infinitely stretchable. We all have snapping points but it's best to prevent that if possible. If you snap, it can take longer to pick up the pieces, so give yourself some breathing space.

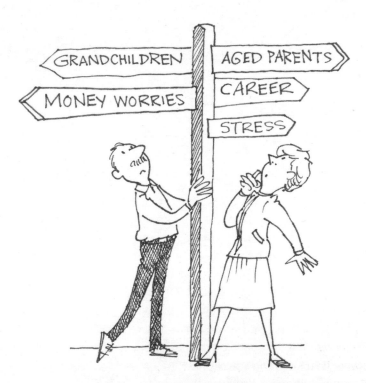

The most important thing to ask yourself is whether you're safe. You will need space and time to sort the situation, but even these will not help if things have got to the danger point already. You may need urgent help that's practical, compassionate and effective. This is especially important if you are responsible for looking after others as well. If you are unsafe (and liable to explode), they will be unsafe too.

If things are so squeezed that your inner being has no space to breath, you need a break. It's right that you do if you feel like this, but make sure you have a safety net and back-up plan, and that anyone you look after has one too. If you are looking after small children – your grandchildren or others perhaps, and you simply cannot manage it one day, you need to be able to say to their parents: 'NO, I'm sorry, I am just too exhausted (or whatever is right) – I can't manage it today', and they need to accept what you say. A similar approach is needed for your other commitments: when you're a carer (see page 171), or a volunteer with a commitment to visiting someone who might be depending on you.

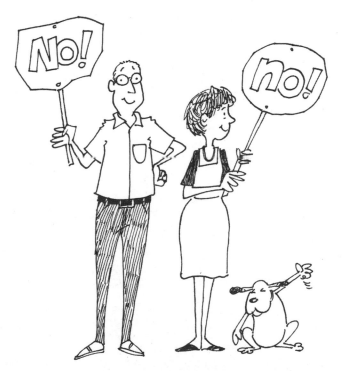

Whatever your situation you should find time now to list your commitments. Flag up for each what the back-up plan is, and ask relevant others to do that too in case there's an emergency.

When you do get space – it's precious. It may be essential for you simply to potter, chill out, with absolutely nothing scheduled but just living the moments. Only you will know what is right. You are the expert on YOU. This is your time, and yours to be. It may be a good time to enjoy doing your mindful breathing, if you haven't been for a while.

If you've managed to rest that's GOOD. Now what do you need to sort out? Have commitments crept up beyond your comfortable capacity? Would less be more? Don't forget, if you're overstretched you may be under-performing – and others may be afraid to say so.

Red flags

- **Alcohol – is it creeping up**? Take action to reduce it, and get help if you need. Drink within safe limits and keep two or more alcohol-free days each week – or stop for a while altogether. Don't drink alone.
- **Are you forgetting important things**? It's a sign you have too many things to attend to. Plan to reduce your stress.
- **Are you crying more, losing interest in sex, not sleeping well**? Are you getting depressed? Do take a breather and see a friend. Sounds as if you need to see your GP. Walk more. Practise your mindful breathing.
- **Are you shouting more**? Sounds as if others may soon be at risk. Take action to reduce the stress, and seek help.
- **Are you staying up later and later to finish stuff**? (Yes, occasionally we all do, but not all the time.)
- **Have you had an avoidable bump in your car**? That's probably the last straw: what more do you need to tell you to get help?

RESOLUTIONS

- ✓ I will keep at least one day a week free of commitments.
- ✓ I will be honest with other people about what I can and can't do.
- ✓ I will take time each day to chill out, even if it's only 20 minutes.
- ✓ I will increase my walking, and breathe mindfully as I do.
- ✓ I will practise mindful breathing for at least 3 minutes every day.

PEARL NO. 10: THE LONG GOODBYE

This technique reduces stress and anxiety with just a few slow breaths. It can stop hyperventilation in its tracks: so use it immediately if you have a panic attack.

✓ With your next breath out: purse your lips gently to make the smallest space between them, and breathe out as slowly as you can. Imagine you're breathing out so gently you would only just make a candle flicker.

✓ Try to make this breath out last as long as you can, aim for 30 seconds.

✓ Then take a gentle breath in through your nose, not a big gasp through your mouth.

✓ Repeat this cycle about ten times. Keep your 'breaths in' small and gentle and though your nose, and keep those 'breaths out' as delicate, quiet and slow as possible.

You may feel that you're about to burst – so great is the urge to rush the breath out. You may not manage 30 seconds straight away. If you do find yourself blowing the breath out in a rush, don't worry: just keep trying, as gently as possible. It will get easier with daily practice. If you play a wind instrument you'll have a head start. When you can make it to 30 seconds, try 45.

Being a carer

This is not about the professional job of caring, which is important and badly underpaid. It's about being an informal, voluntary carer in our 60s and beyond, most often for our next of kin or close relatives. A recent BBC report found that about 1.5 million people over 65 in the UK were carers. One in three people aged 65–74 were caring for someone more than 50 hours a week. This figure rises to over half of people aged 85 and over, among whom the rate is increasing, as the population ages in the UK and in Western society generally.

Being a carer is a challenge that shouldn't be underestimated, however willingly it is taken on. Before you make your decision try to look at what is being asked of you, so you can be really sure you keep control of your own life while providing care for someone you dearly love. A good start is the Carers Direct Helpline: 0300-123-1053, open 7 days a week. And if you are online, www.nhs.uk/conditions/social-care-and-support-guide, gives excellent advice on support, help and carers' rights.

The first thing you must do is ask yourself two very tough questions: 'Do I actually want to be a carer?' and 'Can I manage it?' When you answer you must be true to yourself, and true with yourself – it's not just your life and well-being at stake, it's the life and well-being of the person you care for too.

Caring at home is usually the best option for the cared-for person, whether you are the main carer or not. But sometimes it is impossible, and a nursing or residential home, carefully chosen so that you can visit as often as possible, is the only solution.

If you don't want to be a carer, and know that you can't, then you must not agree to it. It is essential to discuss this with someone who can help you look at other options, for your own health and well-being, but also for the person needing care. If possible (and it isn't always possible), talk to the person you care for, getting someone to be with you if necessary. Make clear that you still love them and they matter to you. Reassure them that you will still be as closely involved as you possibly can, and will want to be.

If you don't want to be a carer, but know that you can *and* that, realistically, there is no other good option, then you may feel you have to make the best of it. So, do all you can to prevent bitterness and resentment. Be sensitive to the fact that care unwillingly offered is almost always felt as such by the person being cared for.

If your answer to the tough questions was a resounding yes, it is essential to plan your caring role so that it enriches the other person but also enables you to live and thrive.

Things to do if you're going ahead

If you have decided to be a carer, contact your local carers' organisation – they can offer valuable support. Here are some other practical suggestions:

- **Inform your GP** about the relevant advanced plans and contingencies. Being a carer will be recorded in your notes to help with your own care.
- **Ask your local Social Services** whether the person you care for needs a care plan, if they haven't got one already.

- **Have enough medication** for the person you care for (and you, if appropriate) in advance of the weekend.
- **Consider a Lion Club green cross sticker** for your front door, flagging up emergency details on your fridge (the message in a bottle project: www.lions105ea.com).
- **Make a back-up plan** for when you are ill – a neighbour, friend or relative.
- **Install a safe key for access**: for other carers, medical, social and emergency staff, in case you're out of the house when they call.
- **Enlist regular visits** from friends known to the person, if they can't organise these themselves – it helps you too.
- **Notify the council**: does it affect your cared one's Council Tax?

ESSENTIAL LIFE SUPPORT FOR CARERS

✓ Keep up your **exercise routine**, eat a **balanced diet**, **sleep** and **keep up your social contacts**.

✓ **Keep a file of all the information you need**: key contacts, supports and resources, medical and medication details of the cared for, copies of advanced plans, and instructions about cardiopulmonary resuscitation, if appropriate.

✓ **Get all the help you can.** If you are the main carer, try to see yourself as a key member of a supportive caring team, rather than just you in isolation. If that is not the reality, how can you bring it about? Your district nurses, GP, local carers group and local social care support can help. So, very often, can friends.

✓ **Be brave; ask for help.** It could be a small thing – a cooked meal once a week, a few hours helping out so that you can go for a refreshing, relaxing walk – it all adds up.

✓ **Empower the one you're caring for** to be as independent as they can. Their independence, however good at the moment or dwindling and slight, is precious to them and invaluable to you.

Planning for the future

Does the concept of **moving on** help you? Can you see something beyond your caring role? Even if it's only planning your annual holiday, have it to look forward to if you can. But plan those daily mini-treats too: the ones your Good Night Thoughts are all about. And for a bit more challenge when (and if) things settle into a pattern, could you keep your hand in with a club or activity outside the home, maybe even a little work: home-based or, ideally, out of it? Have a plan. It helps.

Red flags

If these things are happening, then you're not looking after yourself properly:

- **Increased drinking, smoking or comfort eating**.
- **Poor sleep**, mood dropping, feeling anxious.
- **Feeling angry and bitter**.
- **Shouting at the person you care for** is A DANGER SIGNAL. The person you care for is at risk and you are at breaking point. Talk to family, friends and your GP.
- **Hitting the person you care for** is AN EMERGENCY. This is abuse, and the person you are looking after is being harmed. You are drowning not waving, and the person you are caring for is going to be sinking too. If this has happened, CALL FOR HELP NOW, YOU ARE NO LONGER ABLE TO MANAGE, HOWEVER MUCH YOU THINK YOU CAN. Call your GP or, if you are in touch with a social worker, call them. Otherwise, call a friend and ask them to contact someone for you. Remove yourself from the situation, and find someone to step in as an emergency alternative.

RESOLUTIONS

✓ I will have a daily rest-bit and a daily exercise-bit.

✓ I will have a weekly rest-chunk and a weekly activity-chunk.

✓ I will have a monthly rest-day and monthly interest day.

✓ I will have an annual respite and an annual jaunt away.

✓ I will call friends, family and my GP as appropriate if I see the red flag.

✓ I will call my GP, a neighbour, or a social worker if I realise I have hit the person I care for, and accept I cannot cope.

When dying is on the horizon

Hopefully death is not on the horizon. But you don't need to wait for a terminal diagnosis before thinking about advance decisions (see Chapter 8). It may help you feel more secure about your future, and better able to deal with it when it comes. You may want to discuss organ donation or other plans with your family while emotions are stable.

If you are facing a diagnosis of terminal illness, it usually helps if someone is with you, though it's not always possible. Your reactions may be unpredictable. You may be angry or scared, want to cry or be quite still. It makes a difference if you've thought about the possibility, but it is always unwelcome news and a shock. It usually helps to talk to someone, or know that you can if you need to.

If you are alone, your GP and district nurse team will know about your situation, and want you to feel able to discuss any aspect of it. They can link you to local hospice support services: including Macmillan nurses who can help as part of the caring team around you. If you are approaching death and have few if any family or connections, but do have some savings, think about using some for your care if the time comes when you cannot look after yourself. If you do not have savings, and have a terminal illness, discuss this with your GP and district nurse, who can help you arrange local care for which you may qualify. There may be many sources of help you never had reason to be aware of until now. Don't assume there are none.

If you belong to a church or other group that offers friendly support, don't hide from them. They will want to help in a way that works best for you. Consider letting your priest, minister, rabbi, imam or Elder, or other spiritual guide, know your situation if you are approaching death.

If you know death is not far away, it may be that either because you are naturally sociable or, contrary to all your expectations you want to be now, you become a focus of support for others too. Giving your loved ones permission to ask friends to help might be a breath of fresh air for you and a support for them. You might leave a legacy of new relationships for people who will always treasure your memory.

When you have had some time to adjust to your terminal diagnosis, consider whether any of the following seven special considerations apply to you now:

1. **Do you need to make advance plans now**? Do you want to make a decision against resuscitation should you have a cardiac arrest? If there are no clear instructions and an emergency arises, paramedics may have no choice but to proceed. It may help to discuss this with your GP (see Chapter 8).

2. **Have you made clear whether or not you would like a priest or minister to visit you**? Soon, nearer the time of your dying, or afterwards?

3. **Consider whether your will is in order**. You may prefer your local solicitor to visit you at home to draw up your will, if you feel you cannot do it yourself.

4. **Are you clear about what help and support is available to control pain, sickness or other symptoms**? Is it appropriate to have them to hand now?

5. **Do you have any thoughts about 'assisted dying'?** This is not the same as assisted suicide, which is when someone takes their life without necessarily being terminally ill. Assisted dying is not legal in the UK, but you may have strong views about it, one way or another.

6. **What instructions are there for your funeral**, and who do you want to be informed about your death and the funeral arrangements? Do you have preferences for burial or cremation, or a natural funeral?

7. **Do you want to make clear your views on organ donation**, or even leaving your body for medical research? These are significant personal decisions to make, and though not essential to discuss with others, may be very helpful to.

And then there are the personal, precious things that matter so much:

- **Are there things you really want to do or places you want to visit, before you die**? If so, could you visit them?
- **Are there tasks you really want to finish if you can**, and does that affect the drugs you might be willing, or not, to take? Are there people who could help you complete them, or pick up the torch when you hand it on?

- **What really matters to you now, as you look back over your life and live your days one by one**? Express this somehow, to someone if possible, but put it on paper or screen otherwise, for loved-ones to read when they see you.
- **There are four things that can matter so much to say, and so much to hear**. These are widely recognised since first drawn together by Dr Ira Bryock, a palliative care specialist in the United States, who made a study of what people most wanted to say at the end of their lives: 'I love you', 'I forgive you', 'please forgive me' and 'thank you'.

Bereavement and loss

Loss is painful. Even when you know someone is going to die it can still be a shock when it happens. Some life events have the power to turn our world upside-down by their very nature.

The NHS website (www.nhs.uk) on bereavement is excellent, and discusses in detail what is often involved in accepting the reality of loss, experiencing the pain of grief, adjusting to life, and finally putting less energy into grieving, or moving on.

To begin with, you may not know whether your life will follow the same direction or a new pathway. But the present, however difficult and painful, has to be engaged with in order to be able to face the future, as we saw at the very start of this chapter.

It is a good idea to try to share one's feelings and thoughts, however jumbled, chaotic, contradictory or uncomfortable they may be. If one cannot easily do this with friends or family then it's worth exploring other options. CRUSE Bereavement Care (www.cruse.org.uk) have many local branches and can provide bereavement counselling and support if needed.

There is no rigid progression from one phase of grief to another. All sorts of emotions can well up at different times. Gradually, there are more good days than difficult days. Learning to live with loss is rarely about getting over it, and more about weaving the experience of it, and the memories of the loved one that come to mind, into the fabric of life.

Triggers, like birthdays, the anniversary of the person's death, or the anniversary of special days that marked your relationship, will bring the loss back with a freshness that can be almost overwhelming. It can help to prepare for those times, and have friends or family around you, and perhaps find ways of celebrating your loved one's life with memories that bring joy and gratitude rather than focusing on the pain of loss itself.

It may seem disrespectful to suggest that sometimes even a bit of humour can be good. We usually associate death and loss with tears, but the full humanity of the person who has gone will have been a mix of all sorts of foibles, failures and frustrations, as well as the wonderful things, the strengths, the love and the contributions they have made to your life and others. But laughter can be a form of love and respect, and being able to laugh at the things that are laughable is a tribute to the wholeness of the person who has gone. Laughter is a great healer. Death need not be its great taboo forever. There's a time and a place for all things.

What you can do to come to terms with bereavement and loss

The importance of talking with friends or family as appropriate is difficult to over-emphasise. People will differ in how much they want or need to, and for many picking up the threads of normal life, work and other relationships is the best thing. But most of us need time and talking opportunities. A cup of tea with a friend, a walk through the park with the family, are great ways to work through your feelings.

If you cannot sleep (see page 70) or are finding it difficult to adjust and pick up the threads:

- talk to your GP
- practise mindfulness and other helps (see page 62)
- walk more, especially with friends
- CRUSE can provide helpful support (0844-4779400)

Red flags

It is possible that you are depressed if …

- you are **not eating**
- you are feeling **unremittingly sad** all the time
- you are **waking early and feeling at your blackest**
- you are **losing interest in your appearance and affairs**
- you have **contemplated suicide.**

Call the **Samaritans or your GP right away** if you feel suicidal. When depressed you become unable to do the very things that would help: meet friends, get walking, eat healthily or follow your interests. You may smoke or drink more, getting very unfit. If you, or your family or friends, are concerned about you, please see your GP. Support, talking therapy, and sometimes medication, can help.

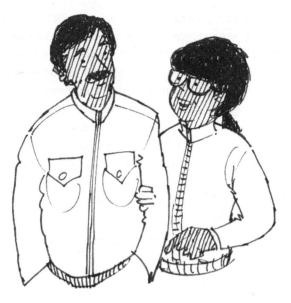

RESOLUTIONS

✓ I will keep in touch with friends and family, keep active and eat healthily.

✓ I will get advice and help, to manage practical affairs, if I need to.

✓ I will see my GP if I can't seem to get on with the normal pattern of life.

Divorce

Facing divorce is not easy. But if it's coming, or has happened to you, it has to be faced. There is excellent help at www.nhs.uk, with seven sensible steps written by a relationship psychotherapist from Relate, Paula Hall. Relate (www.relate.org.uk) is a relationship counselling service offering expert help to couples going through difficult times, including separation and divorce, as well as joint counselling when it is not clear what direction a relationship in distress will go.

Mediation services (see the National Family Mediation, NFM, services at www.nfm.org.uk) may also be very useful. NFM gives online advice about help available, and please check out local mediation services near you if appropriate. These provide specialist lawyers and counsellors trained to help with the complexities of divorce and separation, encouraging a damage limitation approach, especially where there are children to consider. Services may be free, but are usually not.

You need resources and strategies to take care of yourself and protect yourself from harm. But you may also have people who depend on you. If you have children, they will be affected by divorce, however young or old they are. In your 60s, children will be older and often better able to understand. They will want to support both of you, and may feel conflicted and angry. It will be hard for them, and they may need independent support too. There may be grandchildren, who love you both, and are confused about what might be going on, especially if no one has given them a clear explanation they can understand.

There will be practicalities: financial and housing, as well as legal. Working out whether you need professional help, and how to pay for it if you do, is challenging. So it's a triple whammy, however you look at it.

How it feels, and how you face and accept the reality of it, will depend on the circumstances: whether you came to a mutual decision and have been able to plan the steps in a civil and constructive way, with damage-limitation in mind at the start. Or whether it has been one-sided, and you are the one left behind, or the one actively leaving. When communication has been acrimonious, difficult or impossible it is obviously harder, more distressing and potentially more damaging.

It is never too soon to get help: talk to friends, to family and to trusted colleagues. But if you're too dazed and confused to make decisions consider self-referral for talking-based therapy through the NHS and see your GP, to rule out health problems and discuss more immediate support. Facing the reality of divorce means acknowledging there will be a mix of conflicting and intense emotions that need managing.

Trying to understand what happened and how to learn from it can help, but may not be possible immediately. Events may be too hot to handle, and you may only have the energy to manage to keep your head above water initially. But when you can bring yourself to look at the issues and ask why certain critical things happened, it can help you face the present, learn from the past and plan for the future.

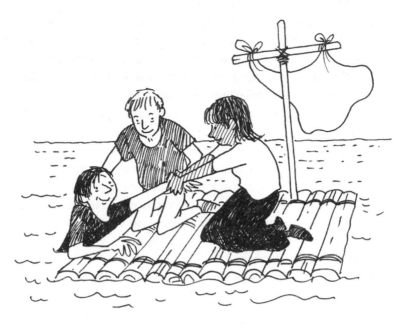

Holding on to your life supports

If you're are going through divorce, you need help to survive now, day by day; help to survive the next few weeks, week by week; and help to get on track for your future. You need to try to point yourself in the right direction for that more distant future even now, when you may not know the exact route you'll take to get there.

If things go badly pear-shaped you need a lifebelt (or two!) to keep you afloat immediately and for as long as you need – some are essential forever (your basics and your friends, in particular), so don't let them go. You need a life raft to clamber onto for a bit more security, just as soon as you can scramble on to it. This will provide your immediate framework for survival over the next few weeks. Then you need your lifeline for the future, to stop you drifting and to keep you in sight of the shore.

Seeing the shore ahead, however distant, will give you a sense of hope and, with that, a greater sense of control.

Hope, and the sense that you are in control of your life, may be in short supply at the moment. You may not need a lifeboat, but it helps to know you can call for one if you do – for example the Samaritans (www. samaritans.org) or 116-123 (in the UK).

So, make a plan for now, a plan for the medium term and a plan for your future.

For now, keep close to your family and friends; eat, sleep, exercise. Focus on the present, don't drink on your own, smoke or comfort eat. Practise mindfulness and avoid negative thinking.

For the medium term, sort out practicalities and priorities for today, tomorrow and next week. Work out how you are going to communicate constructively with your ex, especially if you have children. Be civil if you can. Remember: 'to understand all is to forgive all'. Give yourself, and the other, time, and make your main aim damage limitation – for all concerned. If a relationship has been violent or destructive and it is reasonable not to have direct contact, do consider professional help. This can be useful for discussing general issues that you may need to work through over time, but specifically for advice on making safe contact indirectly, if there is need, for the good of your children.

In terms of your hopes and expectations **for the future** ... this takes time. But as soon as you can, start thinking about it – it's good for you.

Red flags

- Persistent low mood, increased drinking, debt, other people concerned about you? Get help. Talk to friends and colleagues, but see your GP, consider AA, Citizens Advice or a counsellor. And if you're not waving but drowning: call the Samaritans or your GP, ASAP.

RESOLUTIONS

✓ I will keep in touch with my friends.

✓ I will not drink alone.

✓ I will take a day at a time, but think about where I'm heading.

Going it alone

Being single doesn't have to be a problem, and for most of us who are, it isn't. But whether you've always been on your own, or have arrived at being alone through life events: bereavement, separation or divorce, it can be useful to be aware of the risks as well as the benefits of our circumstances.

And a mindful approach to your circumstances, whatever they are, deepens your awareness of them.

So, whatever has been the lead up, where you are now is important and what's on the horizon is interesting, and sometimes useful, to contemplate. The NHS Choices website has an excellent set of pages and links on loneliness in older people.

It's useful to think about because it's clear that being alone can have many pluses. You can make the plans and decisions that matter to you: where you go for holidays, what you do with where you live, when you go out and meet friends, whether you go campaigning or volunteering, or simply going out for a walk in the park exactly when you want.

As we have already discussed, almost everyone will have a range of commitments to other people: organisations, usually a wider family and often your work, all of which you have to juggle with your own particular life choices. Just because you may be alone doesn't mean you have no connections or responsibilities to others.

Of course, being alone can have a darker side too. While it doesn't inevitably lead to loneliness, it is a big risk factor. And loneliness risks yet further loss of social contact, with isolation, depression, increased drinking and ill health. Depression and all its consequences is a vicious spiral, one of the very worst if you don't manage it and roll it back. You need to guard against it, and the best way to guard against it is to counteract it

If loneliness does become a problem don't forget the phone – call a friend, consider getting a pet or offering to take someone's dog for a walk – and meet others doing the same. If you can't think of anyone – think of the Silver Line (started by Esther Rantzen in 2011) on 0800-4-708090, and call them.

What you can do to cope with going it alone

There are three essential ways to help yourself with this issue, all of which you have read about if you've reached this point in the story. **Firstly**, keep your social connections. This is important for everyone, but if you are going it alone, it is the single most important thing. And along with that goes your generous disposition and your capacity to give, in a variety of ways. Giving enriches others, and yourself, a good thing surely?

Secondly, you need to maintain all those activities, physical, mental and emotional, that keep you fit and healthy. You need all the basics of life, but you need to be as physically active as you can, walk more and more quickly, get your sweat up, and strengthen your muscles. It's good for your heart and your joie de vivre. And keeping your mind agile and your brain active is essential for their best working order too.

Don't get fixed in a ruminative past or fixate on an anxious future. You need to learn to live in the fullness of the present, so that learning from the past as well as planning for the future is not, in itself, a burden. And you need to be true to yourself and true with yourself, as well as open to others – who are as complex and contradictory, and sometimes as lovable, as you.

And thirdly, you need your lifebelts, life rafts, lifelines and (hopefully never, but sometimes unavoidably) you need a lifeboat to call. Life is more secure when there are emergency supplies and rescue services to call on should you need them.

Red flags

- **Isolation**: make contact with a friend.
- **Increased drinking**: keep within safe limits; talk to your GP.
- **Depression**: talk to a friend, and discuss with your GP.

RESOLUTIONS

✓ I will keep connected with my nearest and dearest.

✓ I will speak to someone in person or on the phone every day.

✓ I will meet a friend at least twice a week.

Retirement

Many of us retire in our 60s even if we don't do it on our 60th birthday. Increasingly, people work through their 60s and beyond, not least for financial reasons. But if you do retire, it is worth preparing for it if you can. Whatever your future, planning for your retirement is planning for a major life adjustment. It can be many different things: a chance to get on top of the garden, travel a bit, hike or bike with your partner or a new group of friends.

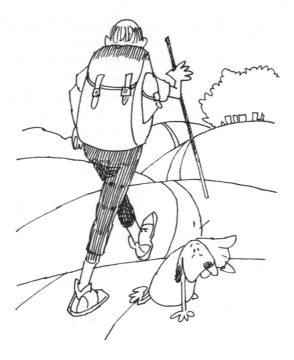

What you can do to prepare for retirement

Many employers, trades unions, bank managers and accountants offer advice on financial planning, especially on pension-related matters. There is good retirement advice online at Age UK (www.ageuk.org.uk). If you have been self employed it can help to have a date for your end-point so you can wind down the number of new jobs you take on.

If you have had a physically active, outdoor job then retirement may reduce the opportunities for exercise and keeping fit. Exactly the reverse may be the case if you've been sedentary. In either case, keep active physically and mentally, have a varied, balanced Mediterranean diet, manage stress, keep connected with others and get rid of harms – with help if necessary – to maintain and improve your fitness and well-being, whatever your future direction.

At home, your retirement is likely to have implications for your partner or spouse. It is a considerable adjustment within a close relationship when one person has been out of the house most of the day, and suddenly is around most of the time. Make time with your partner, to discuss how best to manage the changes. Consider jointly reviewing some of the basics for strong, secure relationships (flip back to Pearl No. 5 on page 56).

If you haven't yet planned a new direction and don't have a clear pattern for your future, it's a big start being aware just how important a purpose in life can be for your self-esteem and self-worth. But if work has been hectic and full on, what you may need most of all is time to re-discover yourself – leaping into new commitments before you are ready may not be wise.

Of course, everyone is different and there is no one size fits all. But having a goal that matters, and engaging in activities that fulfil you, can prevent aimlessness, boredom and low mood.

Red flags

- **Getting isolated, losing daily routines**: get up at the same time each day, join a group or club.
- **Losing fitness**: get walking, join the ramblers club, learn a language.
- **Drinking more:** reduce your intake, count your units, get help for underlying problems.
- **Escalating friction at home:** give each other some space; go for a walk with your partner – air the issues. Consider RELATE, if problems persist.

RESOLUTIONS

✓ I will **do my triple S exercises daily**.

✓ I will **get out of the house every day**, with a plan in mind.

✓ I will **stretch my mind** with new challenges, and keep connected with others.

✓ I will **develop your hobby** or start one, consider volunteering, or a new career.

✓ I will **meet up with other friends** and maintain my connectedness.

✓ I will **work towards a plan** for my direction and goal in life.

✓ I will **be true to myself,** with myself and open to others.

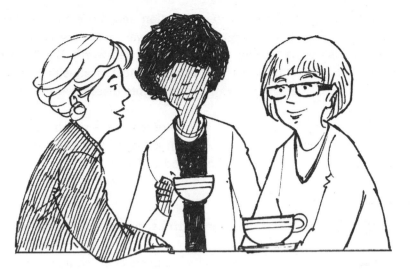

Now here's a big dose of toe-to-top relaxation. It's one of the portable lifebelts we noted at the start. With practice, you will find chunks of time which you least expect, when you can retreat for 15–20 minutes and melt away the tension: muscular and mental. It can also be a good routine when background stress is high, as in some of the scenarios we have looked at above.

PEARL NO. 11: DEEP, DEEP TOE-TO-TOP RELAXATION

This takes about 15 minutes. It is a simple, effective tool for unwinding and relaxing deeply. You can do it for the sheer pleasure of it too!

With each part of your body, this is the cycle. Hold or clench that part of your body as tight as you can for half a minute – and as you tighten the muscles there, concentrate hard on the tension in them. Then, as you relax the part, focus attentively on the soft, relaxed, heavy feel of it. Acknowledge the difference between the tense and the relaxed state of that part of your body.

Find a quiet place on your own, take off your shoes, lie down and close your eyes. With each part of you, repeat the same cycle of tightening and relaxing the muscles focusing on each state while it lasts:

✓ **Toes**: screw them up as tight as you can for 30 seconds, then relax for 30 seconds.

✓ **Knees and calves**: flatten your knees as hard as you can and point your toes towards you, stretching your calves – hold for 30 seconds, then relax for 30 seconds.

✓ **Buttocks**: clench them hard: hold for 30 seconds, then relax for 30 seconds.

✓ **Tummy**: pull in your tummy wall flat: hold for 30 seconds, then relax for 30 seconds.

✓ **Shoulders**: brace them back hard: hold for 30 seconds, then relax for 30 seconds.

✓ **Neck**: thrust your head back into the cushion: hold for 30 seconds, then relax for 30 seconds.

✓ **Eyes**: screw them up tight as you can: hold for 30 seconds, then relax for 30 seconds.

✓ **Jaws**: clench them hard as you can: hold for 30 seconds, then relax for 30 seconds.

✓ **Fists**: clench them as hard as you can: hold for 30 seconds, then relax for 30 seconds.

✓ You have finished the cycle. Lie there and appreciate the relaxation of your body and mind. Rest a few minutes if you can. Then GRADUALLY sit up. WAIT FOR 2 MINUTES, rotating your ankles to get the circulation going, before carefully standing up.

You can use the focused 'tighten and relax' cycle on individual bits of you anywhere, anytime, standing up or sitting down. It can help you relax if you're in a queue, waiting for an appointment, or walking away from an argument.

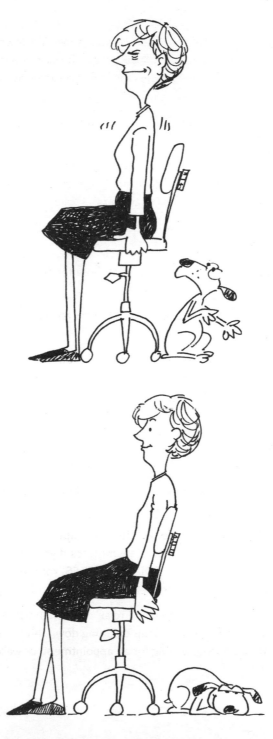

DECISIONS, DECISIONS

Navigating your health care decisions

There's a lot of health care out there. But what you need is appropriate health care for you as an individual. This chapter will help you sort out exactly that. Health needs don't suddenly become different on your 60th birthday, though a few things are set in motion by that happy day, for example, you now qualify for bowel cancer screening.

We'll look at what appropriate care might be – how to steer towards it, and avoid pitfalls, whether from self-care or health-care advice. This means looking at the problems of too much treatment or too little, side effects and harm, bias and sometimes distortion in medical evidence, and how to guard against these.

Armed with all this, we'll look at decision making itself. We'll find it's about balancing benefits and risks, as expected, but also about trust, compassion and accountability within the therapeutic relationship.

Your therapeutic relationships and your decisions
A relationship of equals

At the heart of health-care decisions is a therapeutic relationship. Of course, if it's self-care, it's with yourself. Usually, it will be with your GP, or your consultant, if you have complex medical conditions. In either case, it will be with a health care team as well, working with you and your doctor, to provide you with the best and most appropriate care.

Discussing the benefits and risks of a health-care decision with your doctor, or other health professional, is usually worthwhile. By the time people visit their doctor they have often thought about their problems carefully, discussed them with friends or family and done their own research. This is great if you can do it, as it sets the scene for the perspectives you need to talk about.

And this is a good moment to make an important point. The professional relationship between you and a health care professional (often called a 'therapeutic relationship') is a relationship of equals between you, the expert on you, and your doctor (or other health care professional), the expert in their field.

Your GP is important to you because she or he is usually the coordinator, with you, of your medical care. Your GP usually knows you best, and is familiar with the range of your medical problems and medications. Your consultant is also important and may know you well, but may not be as familiar with other aspects of your history.

Be in charge of your decisions

It is important to be in charge of ALL decisions about your health care if you can, because you are the person who bears the brunt of the outcome for good or ill. Being in control of your own health decisions is important for your well-being. So it is useful to feel as confident as you can about how to weigh up benefits and risks, and evaluate the evidence for treatment.

As well as weighing up your decision to get the right care, you may still want to ask your doctor two famous questions that are often asked:

- **What would you do, doctor?**
- **What would you do *if you were in my shoes*?**

They are slightly different questions, but both good. You may be surprised to hear that studies have shown that asking them is the way most people make their decisions, rather than weighing up benefits and risks. We'll return to the questions again, but they shed light on two aspects of your therapeutic relationships, which strengthen your health care and your decisions about it.

The first thing is the trust, confidentiality, compassion and professional accountability of your therapeutic relationship, which is the basis for good communication and understanding about what really matters to you. The second (to which we will return later) draws attention to advance information you could give your health care team, so they can look at the world as if they were in your shoes – should you be too ill to make decisions yourself at a critical time.

Too much, too little or 'just right' medicine?

There are plenty of good treatments and diagnostic tests and we know how to prevent many illnesses. Much preventable ill health has nothing to do with medicine but with lifestyle, and medicine is there to pick up the pieces when things get broken. But medicine has contributed to preventive health too, vaccinations to prevent infectious disease (see page 210) being the best example. Medical treatments for conditions once thought untreatable: cancer, heart disease and worn out joints, have not only extended life but improved its quality. So we are right to be anxious about losing these advances.

But along with the good has trailed some persisting bad. Not all treatments work and not all tests are necessary. All treatments are associated with potential harms. So in order to weigh their benefits and harms and steer between too much and too little medicine, it is essential to look at what can go wrong.

Work out what matters to you

You may be surprised to hear that more harm happens from over- rather than under-treatment. It hardly seems possible – but it's true. Harm is more often due to side effects or unnecessary treatment, rather than too little care. So we need to avoid too much medicine, but be alert to the possibility of not doing enough when there is something that is right to do.

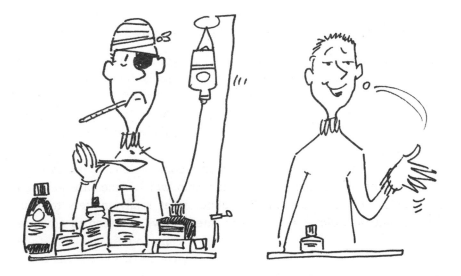

When faced with a health care decision you need to do the following: think hard about what matters to you, ask questions of the experts that are helping you, think carefully about the benefits and downsides and decide on the way forward.

There is no such thing as a wrong problem or a wrong question. What matters is what matters to you. The fact that the problem may become a different beast after discussion, examination, tests or reviews doesn't mean it's not the right starting point. It's YOUR starting point. Nor does it matter if your question isn't the only one that could be asked, or gets replaced by a different one that makes more sense in the light of your discussions.

Isms, attitudinal biases and the risk of under-treatment

The overwhelming tendency in current medicine is too much treatment and this needs to be kept in mind. But under-treatment can happen too, as we saw when considering how many people opt against using hearing aids (see page 97), which would help them.

But there are other causes of under-treatment due to unhelpful attitudes and biases in heath care, and we need to be particularly alert to when they creep in. They're not intended but they can still prevent best care, and until biases are recognised, nothing can be done to overturn them. Making false assumptions that nothing can be done, or worse, that it's not worth doing because of age, gender, or ethnic origin, may lead to under-diagnosis and under-treatment.

It is unlikely you will have met ageism in your 60s. But if you are not called by your proper name, or are referred to as a girl when you're a woman, you'll know to be on the look out for false assumptions about who you are. You are entitled to politely remind people what your name is and what you want to be called.

Terms of endearment in health care (luvvy, dear) are well meant, but usually inappropriate. They can make us feel unseen and patronised, especially unhelpful when decisions are being made or planned. It is respectful, appropriate and empowering to be addressed by the name YOU wish to be called. Equally, if you have a condition such as diabetes, epilepsy or arthritis, you are not the diabetic, the epileptic or the arthritic who happens to be called Mr Sidhu, Ms White and Mrs Cheung. You are Mr Sidhu, Ms White and Mrs Cheung, who happen to have diabetes, epilepsy or arthritis.

Avoiding over-treatment

In order to make the right decisions, you need as much information as possible. Consider the following relevant subjects:

1. **Estimating the benefits and harms of treatments**, not skating over them.
2. Tripping up on **too many medical tests**.
3. **Avoiding lopsided evidence**, which exaggerates the benefits of treatment.
4. **Treatment that isn't really needed**, but just because it's there, and you have a diagnosis, you think you need it.

These things matter to you and to your doctor and are essential to consider in making good decisions.

Getting better estimates of the benefits and harms of treatments

Suppose you were told that a treatment would reduce your risk of a heart attack by 50 per cent. Sounds good, doesn't it? Would you do it? Of course you would. But do you have enough information? Try having a bit more. Which sounds best? Suppose:

- Your risk of a heart attack is **reduced from 4 in 100 to 2 in 100** by treatment, or
- Your risk of a heart attack is **reduced from 4 in 10 to 2 in 10** by treatment.

Heart attacks are always serious events, and your risk of having one is being reduced by 50 per cent in both cases. In each case it is referred to as Relative Risk reduction. But a heart attack is much **less likely** in the first case, and much **more likely** in the second. So Relative Risk is a slippery fish, and needs extra information to be helpful.

You need a ballpark estimate, even if not *exact*, of your actual risk of the problem without treatment, before you can use relative risk reduction to help you make a decision. Using something called the 'Numbers Needed to Treat', or NNTs for short, is a much easier way of talking about the benefit of a treatment.

USING USEFUL NUMBERS: YOUR NNTS

A good way of putting this information together has been developed. It is called the NNT of treatment X:

✓ The **NNT** is the **N**umber of people who **N**eed to be **T**reated with X before the benefit is seen.

✓ So, the smaller the NNT, the better the treatment.

It translates the *relative risk reduction* of a treatment or preventive health step, into the real-life scenario of the *absolute risk reduction*. So, in the example about heart attacks above:

✓ **The NNT is 50 in the first scenario** (the absolute risk is reduced by 2 in 100).

✓ **The NNT is 5 in the second scenario** (the absolute risk is reduced by 2 in 10, or 20 in a 100).

NNTs help most people think more easily about the benefits of a treatment. But you always have to ask yourself 'does this matter' and most importantly 'does this matter TO ME?' A heart attack or a stroke is serious, but a cold or a minor non-cancerous skin blemish is not.

When you finally weigh up your decision about a treatment, whether preventive or curative, you want a high chance of achieving the benefit that matters to you, but also a high chance of avoiding the harm that's important to you to avoid. In other words, the treatment must be likely to be effective enough and safe enough.

Estimating the harms

There are two ways that treatments are associated with side effects:

- **When side effects** *may* **happen**, and their approximate risk is known.
- **When side effects are** *unavoidable,* so need monitoring and managing.

In the first case, where side effects are possible but not inevitable (the majority of treatments), they can be estimated by the NNT approach. In the case of harms, it is the **NNH** that is of interest, where:

- The **NNH** is the **N**umber of people who **N**eed to be treated with X before the **H**arm is seen, and
- **The bigger the NNH, the better the treatment** (because more people can be treated before you find even a single harm).

This is one of the few times when BIGGER IS BETTER – worth making the most of.

So, for effective AND safe treatment you want a low NNT and a high NNH.

The second case, where side effects are unavoidable, is usually found in situations where potent treatment is advised for serious problems that most people would consider **essential** to save life or limb. The treatment **IS** toxic to your body tissue, but **MORE** toxic to the diseased tissue or disease process. For example:

- **Chemotherapy**: for reducing the spread of cancer.
- **Amputation**: life-saving for a gangrenous leg.
- **High dose steroids for saving sight or life**: in severe inflammatory illnesses.

Side effects are unavoidable because of the way the treatment works. But the side effects can be minimised, compensated for and counteracted in various ways.

Chemotherapy is an example where decision making can be very finely balanced. Side effects will vary with the cancer and the chemotherapy. But chemotherapy is getting better and better. It is less prone to side effects than before and there are better ways of managing them. But some side effects usually occur. Most are temporary and manageable, with or without short-term medical help, but they need to be accounted for in decision making.

SUSIE'S LONG-HAUL STRATEGY

Susie was in her 50s and facing breast cancer. She was upset by her diagnosis, but impressed by her 90-year-old mother, who had survived it. She inherited her mother's optimism and straightforward approach to life. Unsure what to do Susie and her partner did research into the issue, had endless discussions with her GP and made her decision to go with chemotherapy. She loved life, and wanted as much of it as she could have. She wasn't going to let a thing like cancer get in her way.

She decided to leave the chemotherapy to her consultants, check in with any side effects that needed action, and DO ALL SHE COULD TO KEEP HERSELF FIT AND BOOST HER WELL-BEING, using complementary medicine and massage for stress relief, and she got a wig to boost her self-confidence. She kept her exercises and her tennis going, just as soon as she had rested from the temporary side effects of chemo, and she ate lots of fruit and vegetables for the best possible dietary variety and balance. She meditated and used mindfulness to help her through the day. She recognised that there would be choppy moments, with tearful and worrying times, and accepted her partner's support and the contact with friends.

She lived as fully as she could through her treatment, being realistic and optimistic, taking charge of her life and steering it, with help from all sides. She did incredibly well, and flourished after her treatment. She was pleased with her health care, and pleased and grateful to her partner, but above all pleased with herself too – she had felt in control.

This story explains why it is critical that you take time to consider what matters to you, what is essential to you, and what is possible for you. Your perspective may not be the same as your neighbour's, your friend's or your family's. Your loved one's feelings and views may be important to include in your decision making, but in the end it HAS TO BE YOUR DECISION.

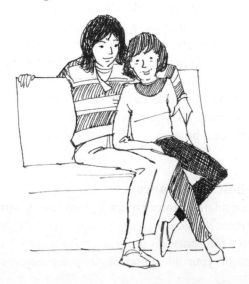

NNT's hidden confusion about risk

When a percentage, say 50 per cent, is given for the probability that a treatment will help, some people think this means it will definitely help, but only by 50 per cent.

What it *usually* means is that some people will be helped, but others won't be. Using numbers needed to treat clarifies this. If the NNT for taking a tablet to reduce your risk of a heart attack is 5, then 1 in 5 people will save themselves from a heart attack, and 4 out of 5 will not. But you don't know whether you'll be the lucky one.

Guestimating if you're the lucky one

This is where you move from the general to the particular – the unique situation with you. This is when you introduce *appropriate* bias. You haven't wanted any bias up to now. What you have wanted is an even playing field, so you can judge whether a treatment works, and how different treatments are rated against each other.

But your unique circumstances: your lifestyle factors, past, family, occupational, allergic and even reproductive history, may all be relevant to the final judgement of whether you are more or less likely to be the one in five lucky winners of the NNT treat.

This is where the joint expertise of you and your doctor, and the confidential, frank and trusting therapeutic relationship need to go FULL THROTTLE. This is where it gets real, for you. It is a critical step in the discussion, so try not to trip over it. There is NEVER certainty, but it is vital to hone the choice to your unique circumstances.

This is also where you introduce your value judgement to the bald numbers. Remember, only you can judge how much achieving the benefit and avoiding the harm will matter to you. This may be the most difficult bit of the whole process. You may want to discuss more, or look online at what others have done in similar circumstances (www.healthtalk.org, or www.patientslikeme.com). Or you may want to dash to that quiet inner sanctum where you can be alone with yourself to think: the bathroom perhaps.

Consider your belt and braces

An NNT of 5 is considered pretty fantastic from the **population health** perspective. Treatment would lead to a phenomenal reduction in illness in the population. From the **individual perspective** it is a big risk reduction. However, in terms of your likelihood of an *individual event*, if you are

ONLY relying on this tablet to help you, you are still more likely to get a heart attack than not. So why rely on tablets alone?

Whether or not you decide to take the tablets (a good example is statins, to reduce the risk of heart attack, see page 108), you know that for many preventable diseases, and for best outcomes in many serious conditions (see Susie's long-haul strategy), taking care of your fitness and well-being MATTERS.

So don't be mean with yourself. Be holistic in your approach: keep fit, reverse the lifestyle causes, bust stress and keep connected. Go for your BBC – your belt and braces control.

Medical tests

There are many different kinds of medical tests and you need to know why a test is being done and how the result might affect your care. A good test is one that tells you what you actually need to know, or rules out something that you need to exclude. Just having tests done without good reason is usually more harmful than helpful. The more tests done, the more likely one will turn out to be abnormal by chance.

Even good tests have limits. All tests need interpreting. Not every abnormal test is significant, though an abnormal result always needs explanation, especially if it has been requested to answer a key question about your care. And to avoid under-treatment, an unexpected normal result needs questions asked too.

Sometimes, test results are misleading, even when technically correct, due to a:

- **false positive result**: suggesting a condition is there when it isn't, or a
- **false negative result**: the condition is there, but doesn't show up.

Screening tests have to meet strict criteria for their false positive and false negative rates, precisely to avoid over-treatment, under-treatment, and all the associated anxiety and cost. A false positive does not mean that the test gave the wrong answer, but that there are other explanations for it being positive rather than the disease in question. A good example of a well-known test that men often think is a screening test for prostate cancer (but isn't) is the so-called **p**rostate **s**pecific **a**ntigen (PSA) test.

THE POINT OF PSA

This is not a good screening test, because it has a high false positive rate. The substance measured (PSA) is very specific for the prostate. But non-cancerous prostate conditions also cause the test to be high, so **it isn't good enough as a screening test for prostate cancer in a population**. But it is a very sensitive test and good for monitoring recurrence of prostate cancer in men who have already had treatment. If you are a man with symptoms suggesting an enlarged prostate, a PSA test may be recommended. However, a raised result may be a false positive, so further tests will be needed for diagnosis.

Avoiding lopsided evidence

Despite all the good medical evidence from carefully planned research, there is still a lot of bad medical evidence. Doctors know this, and are fighting against it, because it usually leads to over-treatment and unnecessary harm.

Evidence-based medicine (EBM) is the key approach. This is co-ordinated by a world-wide network called the Cochrane Collaboration, with scores of teams looking at research publications that make claims for this or that treatment or test, in every field of health and disease. Importantly, it searches for UNPUBLISHED evidence too, which often turns out to be evidence for something *not* working (called, rather confusingly, 'negative results').

Evidence-based v evidence-biased medicine

Evidence-based medicine has found two common problems in research trials and studies (often, but by no means always, drug company based or sponsored):

- **Failure to publish results that do not show the benefit of treatment** (so-called negative results). This is PUBLICATION BIAS.
- **Biased trials**: aka NOT fair tests.

The Cochrane Collaboration insists on fair tests, called randomised controlled trials (RCTs). These are trials where there's always a 'control' group (given an inactive treatment, a placebo, or the usual treatment), so that proper comparisons can be made with the new treatment of interest. Critically, participants are randomly distributed between the control and the treatment groups – so bias isn't built in from the start. Even better is the 'double-blinded' RCT (not always possible), where neither participants nor researchers know who's had what, so the results have to speak for themselves.

In the All Trials Campaign, launched in 2013, the Cochrane Collaboration called for the publication of ALL results (negative and positive) from trials, whether of drugs or other treatments. It's usually only the 'success' stories that get publicity. EBM works to change that.

EBM has developed research to put ALL the evidence together: super big studies called meta-analyses. These bring together the results of ALL the good quality RCTs of a particular treatment, whether they show the treatment works or not. If lots of different studies from different research groups all point in the same direction, it makes it less likely that a finding is due to chance alone. By the same token, if the results from different studies pull in different directions, with results across the studies cancelling each other out, it makes it much less likely that the positive findings in a few groups are real (or apply to everyone). However, researchers have to be very careful. Occasionally, there are important reasons why study results cancel each other out, and if the research topic is very important, more studies may be needed before dismissing treatment X as ineffective.

But there's resistance to EBM. The commercial interests of drug companies sometimes actively work against the release of negative results, and influence the general public, the medical profession and sometimes governments, by pressure from advertising, lobbying and sponsorship.

So there is still reluctance from some doctors to stop treatments even when they're proved not to work, because they're so used to prescribing them. The obvious example is antibiotics for viral infections like heavy head colds, most sore throats, and acute bronchitis – which are usually viral.

Countering the resistance are: NICE (**N**ational **I**nstitute for Health and **C**are **E**xcellence) Guidelines for Treatment, which is NOT DRUG COMPANY SPONSORED; the Cochrane Collaboration's All Trials register, and the James Lind Library, which is online and in the public domain.

The growth of evidence-based medicine has transformed the approach of most health professionals working with you to help you make the right decisions for your care. However, there's still a long way to go.

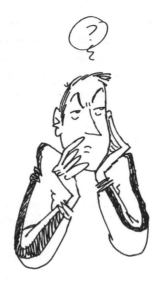

**YOUR RESEARCH: YOUR BRAIN AND
OTHER INTELLIGENCES**

1. **Keep focused** on what matters to you.

2. **Think about your own experience**: what can you learn from it?

3. **Be suspicious of websites full of commercial advertising** or wanting your money, they have vested interests and will be biased.

4. **Go to good sources**: the NHS Knowledge website at www.nhs.uk gives clear, evidence-based information; Medline Plus, at www.nlm.nih.gov/medlineplus, from the National Library of Medicine in the United States; The Cochrane Library of Evidence Based Medicine at www.cochranelibrary.com. The James Lind Library at www.jameslindlibrary.org, gives illustrated information on landmarks in the use of fair tests, and information about pitfalls and biases in medical treatments; Health Talk (www.healthtalk.org) is a continuing collection of people's experiences living with different health conditions, reflecting on the health care they have received – and what they found helpful or not; www.patientslikeme.com, is another useful site.

Treatments that aren't really needed

There are so many treatments and tests that it's tempting to reach for them when they're not needed. Here are seven common types of unnecessary treatments and tests:

1. **Treatments that aren't essential** – and can go wrong, even in the best hands.
2. **Treatments that don't work** – and cause unnecessary harms, avoid them.
3. **Existing treatment that's not properly used** – you need help to use it, not more treatment.
4. **Too much treatment already** – the problems may be due to its side effects.
5. **It's not medical treatment**, but a different approach, that's needed.
6. **Lifestyle, not disease, may be the problem** – treatments may miss the point.
7. Asking for **tests that don't answer the question** you need to ask.

It is often the case that the best way to solve the problem bothering you is not a medical approach at all. And if you do opt for treatment, it's rarely the only thing worth putting a bet on, as we have discussed already. Almost always, keeping as fit as you can will be important too.

Success can never be completely guaranteed or harm ruled out. So it's time well spent deciding whether a treatment is really essential to you, before inviting even a small risk of harm. This is why you have to sign an informed consent before you go ahead with any surgery.

Joint replacement surgery for the knee can be a very good operation if you really need it. But if another way of solving your knee pain was a trial of weight loss, physiotherapy and getting more active, then it may be premature to think of it. And the outcome (if you eventually needed surgery) might be much better if you did shift that extra half a stone (just over 3 kilograms) first.

But deciding whether or not a treatment or procedure is essential depends on context, and needs careful judgement.

CONTEXT MATTERS

You always have to weigh up decisions in context to do the right thing for you given the circumstances. Sometimes, decisions are finely balanced.

For example:

✓ **An operation to remove a bowel cancer** is usually considered essential, especially if caught early. However, there could be wisdom in **declining** surgery if you only had a few weeks of life ahead and wanted to spend them with your family, doing things that really mattered to you, rather than recuperating from an operation.

✓ **Cardio-pulmonary resuscitation (CPR) has a high chance of failure**, but is always worth trying, to save life, UNLESS a person has specifically said they don't want it given certain circumstances (see page 176).

✓ **Cosmetic operations**, including breast implants, may be very difficult to decide upon. The outcome may be worse than before and the operation may not be essential. But a good result may transform your self-esteem.

✓ **An operation to remove a cataract** may or may not help (if your vision is poor for other reasons, it may not add much, and can go wrong). If it is essential to drive, it may be essential to have surgery. But this is not always the case, and the possibility of harm needs considering.

HRT effectively controls menopausal symptoms, but is associated with an increased risk of breast cancer and heart disease – depending on the type of HRT. **But context still matters**. Detailed risks and benefits for different HRT are given in 2015 NICE guidelines (www.nice.org.uk), and for some women, the balance of benefits and risks of certain types of HRT may be acceptable.

And then there's treatment that doesn't work (see below). Optimism is a good approach to life and to health care, but **over optimism** when treatment doesn't really work, will lead to harm simply by introducing unnecessary risk. Evidence presented for the benefits of treatment or tests may be unintentionally over-inflated and the risks minimised (see page 20).

An example of treatment that doesn't usually work well is 'knee-washout' (using keyhole surgery) to flush out osteoarthritis debris from a painful knee joint. Keyhole surgery for the knee works well for problems like repairing ligaments or removing a torn cartilage, but not for washing out debris.

When you have moved from the stage of defining your problem to the stage of a possible planned surgical operation, it is wise to ask:

- **What is the usual success rate?** Ask your GP, consultant, or look online.
- **What is the local success rate, at my hospital?** Ask your GP, your consultant, or look online.
- **On balance, is it worth me going ahead?**

Your balancing exercise: the decision-making one

At some point, a decision has to be made, even if it's an informed decision to postpone until you are more certain. If it is an urgent decision and you can't think clearly, then it is your doctor's duty to make it on your behalf, with your permission and all the necessary input from those who know you well.

But, assuming you can and want to be in control of your decision, this is the time to weigh up what is right for you.

The decision ahead of you is likely to be: do I watch and wait? Do I go ahead with treatment? Or, if it's essential to do something: which of X, Y or Z should I do?

Your reflections

You need time to focus on making your decision. It may be helpful to go for a walk, and practise your mindful breathing. Whether or not it's a life-changing decision, you want to get it right if you can – so give it all the time you need. You may want to jot your thoughts down on paper or screen, as you weigh up what really matters.

You'll need to think about whether you would blame yourself – or someone else – if it did go wrong. You need to ask yourself if it's the right time for you to have treatment, and where to have it, particularly if it's an operation with a need to convalesce afterwards.

If possible, sleep on your decision before you talk to anyone else about it again. You know you, and whether or not you DO need to talk to someone again at this point. But it's a vulnerable time, when it might be easy for someone, with good intention, to derail you from your best judgement about what is right for you. See how you feel in the morning, and what your decision looks like to you then.

Don't be afraid that you have irrevocably missed out if you decide to watch and wait. PROVIDED YOU AND YOUR DOCTOR HAVE EXCLUDED RED FLAGS, it's rarely the case that you have, and it's often a good policy, if well informed and carefully thought about.

MINDFUL WATCHING AND WAITING: THE SAFE WAY

If you come to a mindful decision to watch-and-wait it means you have asked the final key question and given your answer:

✓ The question: does watching and waiting warrant the small risk of harm?

✓ Your answer: Yes, it does.

So, to make your watchful waiting safe:

✓ Always have a safety net.

✓ Know who to call if things get worse.

Discuss with your doctor very specifically what you need to watch out for. For example, if you have an ulcer that's appeared on your tongue, it may be a harmless 'aphthous' ulcer, which usually goes in about 10 days or so. But if it doesn't, or is getting bigger, you need to report back to your doctor or dentist without fail.

So if things don't get better, or events happen that worry you, then you need to review them **as appropriate – and** you need to know with whom. It is usually your GP, but it might be your practice nurse, pharmacist, hospital consultant, optician or dentist – depending on the problem.

When you simply cannot decide what to do

If, at the end of the day you cannot decide what to do, *you*, the expert on you, may need to go back to your expert health professional – usually your doctor, and ask those two famous questions again, if you haven't done so already:

- **'What would you do, doctor?'** and
- **'What would you do *if you were in my shoes*?'**

You may not need or want to, but if you do, you should and can. This is the level of trust you should expect to be able to have with your doctor, either your GP, who is likely to know you best, or your specialist if it's a decision best shared with them. Or both.

But even if it is not a doctor who knows you, it is your right to expect that any doctor, or health-care team, will do the very best they can for you, as if they were seeing the situation from your perspective and standing in your shoes. You may be seriously ill, or even unconscious. The therapeutic relationship is *intended* to cover these very possibilities, and is geared towards doing the very best for you, as far as is possible.

And here is a puzzle that you yourself can solve in advance. How can a health-care team be sure they are acting not just in your best interests, but as if they were in your shoes? There are three things that you could help them with:

1. **Advance plans for special circumstances** when you cannot make decisions.
2. **Contact numbers for significant people** in your life who could advise.
3. **Access to key information** in your medical notes.

It is now possible for your GP, with your permission, to share crucial information that you agree to share (medication, allergies, significant past or present medical history, **advance plans**) with hospital medical teams, via the NHS secure information highway (the NHS Spine). You may not want to do this and can opt out of it. But it is a good way of helping heath-care teams do the best for you.

If you are conscious and able, and have asked your doctor what they would do in your shoes, you still have to decide whether or not to accept this advice – because you are the one who has to agree to proceed, or not, with the treatment.

The ball's in your court.

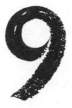

9

HEALTH CARE: CHOOSING AND USING IT WISELY

There are different kinds of health care each with its own particular decisions. One is to do with medical problems and ongoing medical conditions. Another is whether or not to take preventive health measures: from lifestyle changes, to vaccinations, to screening tests that operate at population level, which you will be invited for unless you choose to opt out. Yet another is presented by the fact that each of us, one day, will die. And some of us, sadly, will lose our capacity to make fully informed decisions in our extreme old age or earlier, because of dementia or other issues.

Health care is about preventing problems and shrinking them as much as possible if you have them. Sometimes taking care of problems makes them disappear, but appropriate care is always about making them more manageable and less intrusive. However big problems may seem from one perspective, they can be shrunk so that living your life is the most important thing.

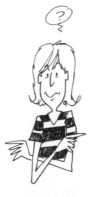

We'll look at preventing disease first – vaccinations against common, serious infections, and lowering your risk of non-infectious diseases by lifestyle changes and appropriate health checks.

Then we'll examine the so-called preventive health services. In reality, they are early detection and problem-shrinking services. They respond to early signs of serious disease, pick them up at regular checks or hunt them out by screening people at increased risk (whole populations by age and sex, if needed). But you have to choose to opt in or out of them. Early detection – what screening is all about – can often lead to cure or more effective treatment and prevention of more serious disease later on.

Living well with continuing conditions is also about shrinking their impact, by managing them appropriately and building up your fitness and resilience despite them.

Self-care and health care to prevent serious disease

Prevention should ALWAYS be better than cure because if it isn't, it isn't worth it. Preventive health measures are recommended when the best evidence suggests that two things are true:

- **The problem is serious and common** enough to take preventive steps.
- **The preventive step has only a small risk** of harm for the majority of people.

Judgements about the **likely** benefits of preventive health are usually made at population level. They are important because they mean that the overwhelming likelihood is that you will benefit from prevention.

But it will always be necessary to check that the general truth applies to you as an individual, on every occasion. So preventive care is ALWAYS a mix of self-care and health care. For example, if you are severely allergic to part of a vaccine, you shouldn't have it. Similarly, you will need to ask yourself questions about your safety to exercise and, if you have medical conditions you may need advice too.

Reducing your risk of infectious disease by vaccination

After pure, clean, running water and a sewage system separate from it, vaccination (or immunisation) is the most cost-effective way of preventing infectious disease.

Vaccination works by boosting your resistance to bacteria or viruses very specifically, and sometimes by contributing to herd immunity (when enough people are vaccinated that transmission is reduced or stopped altogether).

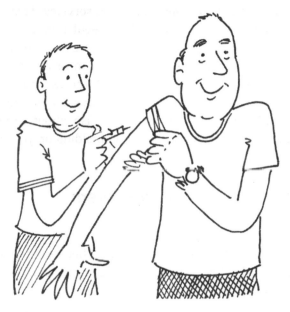

Isn't basic good health, hygiene and occasional medication enough?

It's true that having a healthy balanced diet and the simple but effective health and hygiene step of washing your hands boosts your basic resistance to infection, and helps break the chain of infection and transmission. Always consider condoms if you're sexually active, and if you are recommended to take anti-malarials when travelling abroad, and you're not allergic to them or likely to have an adverse reaction, it is wise to take them.

But it's not always enough. Pandemic flu, which swept the world in the early 20th century, killed millions, including the young and healthy. The World Health Organization (WHO) has a race against time each year to update the flu vaccine, to protect us against newly emerged strains. Older people, and those with significant conditions at any age, are highly susceptible to the complications of flu. So immunisation is worthwhile.

New infections emerge, and old ones step in when immunity drops or antibiotics are used too much. Germs multiply and mutate rapidly, evolving much quicker than we do. They become resistant to antibiotics and anti-virals and may even (in the case of influenza virus) evolve vaccine-resistant strains.

Those of us in our 50s and 60s grew up confident that infectious disease was cracked – after all, smallpox had been eradicated by vaccination (the first example of the use of the term). We believed antibiotics, and more recently anti-virals, would always be there to fight infection. But we have had to adjust to a different reality.

We know that antibiotics can be lifesaving when used carefully. It's not an exaggeration to say that they have enabled safe, life-changing operations we take for granted: joint replacements, abdominal surgery and organ transplants. But the overuse of antibiotics for trivial symptoms, like coughs and colds, has been bought at the price of bugs resistant to their use when it really matters.

We have to stay one step ahead of the game with germs. We need to prevent them infecting us where possible and use the treatments we have much more wisely and selectively. So vaccines have a very important place.

Can everyone have vaccines?

The majority of people can have the majority of vaccines. But occasionally they cannot, and this is why questions are always asked individually before vaccinations are given.

If someone has a genuine egg allergy they need to avoid flu vaccines, which are grown on eggs. Another example is that immunosuppressed people cannot have so-called live vaccines (for example, the shingles vaccine). In such people the weakened vaccine strains will multiply more and this might cause harm.

Here's a list of vaccinations to expect in your 60s:

- The influenza shot.
- The common pneumonia shot.
- Basic vaccination courses (or outstanding boosters) if still needed: tetanus, whooping cough, diphtheria, MMR.
- Travel shots, where indicated.
- Hepatitis B: if indicated for occupational, lifestyle, or volunteering (those that may bring you into contact with other people's body fluids, such as the medical or nursing profession).
- Shingles: (this is offered from age 70, so only if you are 69 now).

The influenza virus is the greatest escapologist of all time – the Great Houdini of infectious disease. Influenza can kill. When it does it is usually because people have inadequate immunity to it. It can cause inflammation in the lungs, making them congested, which strains the heart and often paves the way for severe bacterial pneumonia. Even without complications influenza can flatten you for many days.

The flu vaccine is still an injection into your upper arm. It is not a live vaccine so cannot give you flu. Occasionally, it gives you a slightly sore arm or a mild fever as the immune response is activated. A new, live, highly effective nasal spray vaccine has recently been introduced for small children and, in time, may be used for adults.

An annual flu shot is recommended if you:

- are 65 or over
- have diabetes, heart disease, asthma and other chronic lung disease, kidney disease, disabling neurological disease, cancer or had your spleen removed
- are immunosuppressed due to HIV, chemotherapy and certain other drugs
- live in a residential home
- are a carer.

Even if you are not yet 65 and have no significant medical condition, it is still reasonable to weigh up the benefits and risks of an annual flu shot as it is licensed for use in adults of whatever age, and available in many pharmacies after discussion with the pharmacist (and the GP if necessary).

Reducing your risk of non-infectious disease with self-help

Throughout this book we have looked at the lifestyle changes that can increase your fitness, improve your well-being, build your resilience and at the same time reduce your risk of many preventable diseases. To recap, you can reduce your risk of all of the major diseases including heart disease, type 2 diabetes, stroke, many cancers, kidney failure, depression, cirrhosis of the liver, digestive problems and some dementia if you:

- **get** physically and mentally **active**
- find and keep your **healthy weight**
- adopt a **Mediterranean diet**
- **stop smoking** and keep your **alcohol intake in safe limits**
- build and maintain your **connectedness with others**
- keep your **blood pressure under control**
- **bust stress, practise mindfulness, share happiness** and **be true to yourself**.

Walking is one of the best things you can do, but discuss it with your GP first if you're not sure. If you haven't had your blood pressure or pulse checked in years, it's a good idea to check these, and ALWAYS report a suspected irregular pulse.

Preventive health services

These are designed to pick up and, if necessary treat, early signs or increased risk of serious diseases. It's about 'a stitch in time' to save things unravelling later, and includes prompt responses to your red flags, routine screening services and opportunistic screening.

Prompt response to your red flags

The free NHS health check: five yearly from age 40-74, helps reduce the risk of heart disease, stroke, type 2 diabetes, kidney disease and vascular dementia. It detects high blood pressure, excess weight, discusses smoking, alcohol use and level of activity, and checks your cholesterol. It allows your risk of heart disease (your Q-risk) to be calculated and, if necessary, a discussion about statins for prevention.

If you are at high risk of osteoporosis it is important to pick this up, so you can take action to reduce your risk and prevent a hip or spinal fracture. Why not check out your own FRAX assessment at NHS choices, on www. nhs.uk - and follow it up!

Screening programmes

Your decision to opt in or out of screening programmes will depend on weighing up the balance between early detection and its advantages, and the small increased risk of anxiety, over-treatment due to false positives and potential under-treatment due to occasional missed disease. If you have opted out of important routine screening your GP is usually informed, so you can both be extra vigilant for early red flags suggesting serious disease.

The main screening programmes in your sixties are for cervical cancer, breast cancer and fragility fractures in women, abdominal aortic aneurysm in men and colon cancer in everyone.

Opportunity-based screening

Opticians may pick up macular degeneration, glaucoma or evidence of diabetes, high blood pressure or other problems affecting your eyes. Dental checks may pick up mouth cancer. Continuing condition reviews screen for depression. Every GP (and nurse) consultation is an opportunity to spot a red flag and bring it to your attention for action.

Individual screening for increased risk of disease

This may not be one of the main screening programmes, but appropriate for you if you have a family history of certain conditions. For example: glaucoma (annually, rather than just at the routine eye checks), multiple colon polyps by colonoscopy, high risk of certain groups of cancers, or certain kinds of heart disease, and other very rare conditions. This individually tailored screening is offered within the NHS.

SCREENING YOUR HOME HEALTH

The number one offender is your medicine cabinet. It may be a historical record, an art installation, or a convenient mirror for your daily shave. But if it isn't up to date, it's a health hazard – for you in the dark, and inquisitive grandchildren at any time. Chuck out ALL out-of-date and unnecessary medicines, especially ALL unused antibiotics (unless you have special instructions). You have been warned. Keep it high on the wall and preferably locked, so tiny fingers cannot reach it.

While you are at it, here are some other domestic matters to consider:

✓ Do you have a carbon monoxide monitor? If you have a gas boiler it's recommended.

✓ Are your electrics in safe working order?

✓ Sort out slip mats, loose steps and wobbly handrails to reduce the risk of falls.

✓ If you are living alone, do you have a chain and a spy-hole on your front door?

✓ Do you have a good torch ready in case of power cuts?

✓ Do you have a bag of frozen peas in the freezer for minor injuries?

✓ Do you have a first aid box handy?

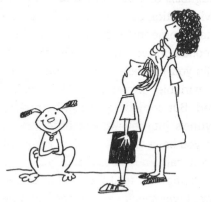

Living well with continuing conditions

These are conditions likely to need managing for the rest of your life: coronary heart disease, high blood pressure, type 2 diabetes, inflammatory bowel disease, asthma, some kidney disease, epilepsy, certain other neurological disorders, and many mental health problems. A study in 2012 of the Scottish population showed that half of 50-year-olds had at least one long-term condition and, by age 65, almost all had more than one.

Actively fostering your healthy lifestyle will not only improve how you feel now, it can help reduce the risk of complications of these conditions, and contribute directly to their good management. Sometimes, finding your healthy weight and keeping as fit as possible can even roll them back, as has been found with type 2 diabetes. Practising mindfulness reduces the rate of recurrence of depression, to name just two examples.

It would be naive and wrong to pretend these conditions never affect your quality of life – they can, even when best managed. This is one reason why depression occurs quite frequently in people with continuing conditions, and is routinely asked about at your reviews. You need some luck to avoid complications, but you can *feed* good luck with your lifestyle to a large extent.

Other long term conditions

There are other kinds of long-term conditions one of which is cancer, an umbrella term for many different types which behave very differently. Others are progressive conditions for example Parkinson's disease, or dementia.

If you have Parkinson's disease, your medication schedules need careful timing and tuning. Knowing what matters to you is essential.

If you have a diagnosis of early dementia, you need closely integrated care and support. Medication can sometimes help, so discuss it with your doctor and always take someone with you if you can.

Whatever your condition, you will benefit from a healthy lifestyle with activity appropriate for you, mental and social stimulation, and plenty of treats!

Cancer is very variable. Increasingly it is picked up early, treated effectively and cured. But sometimes it can be progressive and terminal. With cancer, everyone's journey will be different and require different support and care. If you have cancer, it still applies that a healthy lifestyle, keeping as fit as you can and maintaining your social connectedness, is important to well-being and to the outcome of the cancer itself. This holistic approach, whatever specific treatment might be needed, is strongly endorsed by the Macmillan Foundation – experts in the care and support of people with cancer.

Coping with the shock of a serious disease, whether cancer or one of the more progressive conditions, will need support: from your GP, consultant, specialist nurse, support groups and services offered for the specific conditions: www.parkinsons.org.uk, www.alzheimers.org.uk, www.macmillan.org.uk.

Useful approaches to your continuing health care

In your 60s it is wise to think about advance plans for your health care should you be too unwell to make decisions in the future. Having a condition, especially a very unwelcome one like cancer or a progressive disease, may make this even more relevant (see page 221).

If you have a condition or are diagnosed with one there are several golden rules:

- **Limit the damage** straight away; respond to red flags and warnings.
- **Stabilise the condition** to contain it, but if beyond your control, get help.
- **Keep it controlled**, know what to watch for and what to put in place.
- **Shrink the condition** as much as possible (see page 209).

We only need to look around at our family and friends to find inspiration from others who have been able to shrink down their problems.

THE SHRINKING MACHINE

When you develop a condition that's not going away any time soon, shrink it as small as possible. Shrink the condition in five directions ...

1. Try to **make it disappear** (can it be cured?).

2. Try to **reverse it** (overweight, metabolic syndrome).

3. Try to **make it as small as possible** (build up your strengths).

4. Try to **slow it down** (keep as fit as you can).

5. Try to **prevent it taking over your life**.

... and with seven steps:

1. **Go for a cure if possible**: why not lose excess weight and aim to cure your type 2 diabetes. You may need your medication for a while, but you may reach a point when you don't. Increasingly, cancer is curable, and when it isn't can often be well managed with appropriate treatment and support.

2. **Remove the causes**: get help with problem drinking; divorce those ciggies.

3. **Reverse the causes**: find your healthy weight, and improve your metabolic health and painful arthritic knees at the same time; and STOP WEARING SHOES THAT PINCH YOUR FEET.

4. **Build up the other parts of you**: keeping fit boosts your well-being and reduces complications in most continuing conditions.

5. **Compensate for loss of function**: for goodness sake, consider a hearing aid if you need one. And a good prosthesis after an amputated lower leg can restore your mobility.

6. **Prevent illness returning**: practise mindfulness, keep connected with others and take regular exercise to keep depression at bay. Minimise harm from overtreatment: scrutinise your medication

regularly with your pharmacist and GP, and report side effects promptly. Bring your mindful, evidence-based research to all your health-care decisions (see page 203).

7. **Prevent it taking over your life**: pick up that hobby again.

This is about taking care of your body when it's not working so well. As always, you need the foundations of physical, mental and emotional fitness, and all your social supports and interests: in other words the rich context of your life. But you also need to look at particular aspects of your lifestyle that need special focus given your condition, as well as the medical focus directed at keeping your condition under control.

You, your primary health care team (GP, practice and district nurses, therapists and receptionists), local pharmacist, hospital consultant and specialist nurses (if you have any), are all part of this endeavour. But you are the key person, and with your GP, are the key coordinators of your care.

Continuing care reviews

There are many different kinds of health care appointments, and it can save time and frustration when everyone knows what to expect. If you've been asked to make an appointment, check its purpose beforehand to make sure you need it. If it's a regular review to discuss your condition, key questions to ask (apart from reviewing the condition itself) are whether you are getting too much or too little medicine and what advice you need to keep as fit and active as you can? If these questions cannot be addressed at your review, find an opportunity to discuss them as soon as possible.

If you have several conditions, is it worth trying to streamline your appointments? The annual review of your main condition is a great opportunity for information sharing and looking at what's critical to your progress and well-being. What you cover will vary according to the nature of the problem, and who is reviewing it with you. Depression is common, and your mood and well-being should *always* be enquired about.

Go to your various appointments armed with your urine sample, log books and medications to discuss as appropriate. Sometimes, making a separate appointment from your annual review allows you time to discuss other worries about your condition.

Medication reviews are also important, the more tablets you take the more likely you are to have problems from side effects. Prescribed medicines can be beneficial, but some cause falls, nausea, diarrhoea, stomach bleeding, constipation and, when taken long-term, dependency – even though the original need has gone. Your GP will be keen to help you stop medication you no longer need. The major culprits are likely to be codeine-based painkillers, sleeping tablets and tablets to relax you, which should be used for the shortest period possible.

If you have many conditions and it is *essential* to be on several different medications, discuss with your pharmacist having them in a weekly box system (often called a dosset or nomad system) to make it easier to remember what to take. And if you are partially sighted, or have arthritis of your hands, do mention this to the pharmacist who will want to help you accordingly.

Prescribed drugs and your brain

There is concern that some older types of sedating antihistamines, antidepressants and bladder stabilising medications may, over time, affect your brain function. If you are worried about this, check with your pharmacist and doctor – **please don't stop anything** without discussing it with one of them first. But provided you have what is essential, less is usually more when it comes to medicines.

Complementary health care

Complementary health care often sits happily alongside orthodox care. Susie's example in the last chapter showed this, when she opted for chemotherapy (standard, evidence-based treatment for her cancer), but also decided that complementary therapy, including a new diet, massage and other approaches, would help her well-being meanwhile. So a wise approach might be to **use the orthodox, evidence-based treatment for a serious condition**, but add other things in if you want.

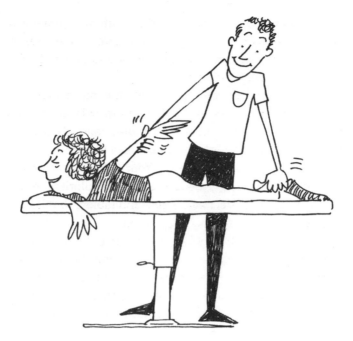

There are plenty of widely practised complementary approaches, such as acupuncture, chiropractice, osteopathy, massage (check with your oncologist if you have cancer or have chemotherapy planned: usually it's fine, but occasionally you may be advised against it), aromatherapy and others. When done carefully by trained practitioners, they don't often cause harm and can help. They allow for something that has declined, understandably but lamentably in many ways, **the human touch**.

Advance planning

Advanced plans are arrangements you might want to put in place should you be unable to make decisions for yourself in the future. Three important legal arrangements you can make are your **last will and testament**, **advanced decisions** (aka Advanced Directives), and a **lasting power of attorney**. Written documents **without** legal status are known as advanced statements, and can guide people about your general wishes: for example whether or not you would want to be looked after in a nursing home, but they are not legally binding. NHS Choices gives basic advice (www.nhs.uk).

Your **will** details how your estate and possessions should be divided between your beneficiaries. You can get advice and download wills from the WHICH website (www.wills.which.co.uk) with instructions for completion, but it points out that if your affairs are complex, it is wise to seek a solicitor's advice.

Advance decisions are legal documents, which specify (for example) whether or not you would want life-sustaining/supporting treatments given certain circumstances. The documents must be signed, witnessed and dated appropriately to ensure they are legally binding (as with your will), but you don't need a solicitor. Forms can be downloaded with instructions from, for example, www.mydirectives.com.

There are two sorts of **lasting power of attorney** (LPA), granted when you appoint someone to act on your behalf about matters of property and finance, or in your best interest in matters of your health and welfare (as if they were in your shoes) – or both.

They are separate applications, even if the same person is appointed to do each task, and you need a solicitor to set it up. The Alzheimer's Society has an excellent website covering both sorts of LPA (www.alzheimers.org.uk).

You don't have to be 60 to plan ahead, any adult over the age of 18 who is mentally capable can make advanced decisions. But if you have a serious and potentially life-threatening illness, or several conditions any of which could suddenly become worse, it is sensible. It is often as much to help and guide those you love, who will want to act in your best interests and may be anxious about how best to do it, as it will be to guard your own well-being. It is not just dementia that can render us mentally incapable of making major decisions – accidents affecting our consciousness or sudden events like stroke can too, temporarily or permanently.

The important thing is to get your plans out of your head (where no one else can see them) and onto paper, or better still online (for example, at www.mydirectives.com), so they can be referred to if necessary – whatever happens to you (or your property) and wherever you are. They can be updated as and when you choose.

It's a good idea to discuss important matters concerning your future health and welfare with those you trust and love. But remember, it's you, unpressured by others, who must make the final choices about what you would want as guiding principles for your care. So it's worth thinking carefully about what matters to you, and talking to your GP can be helpful when it comes to significant advance decisions affecting your life and health.

Take care of the whole of you – it's all yours

It's time to put it all together. You are the specialist, the worker and creator of your own care. You are the mistress or the master of your ship. Make a date with yourself from time to time, and review You. How about New Year's resolutions and half-yearly reviews? We (the authors) are lucky. We have summer solstice birthdays. Which means we can have New Year's resolutions *and* half-yearly reviews nicely timed to our birthdays. But you don't need a birthday to look at where you are and how you are. The solstice rises for everyone. And no, you don't have to be a druid or a hippy (but those were the days my friend).

When you meet up with yourself for your review, have four Ps up your sleeve:

1. Prevention
2. Protection
3. Picking things up early
4. Prompt action

You know you. Taking stock once a year may be quite enough. But if you've got a fair way to go to regain your fitness, a half-yearly review may be a good plan. And if you're living full pelt, pulled in all directions, scarcely able to stand still and collapsing into bed for your only rest: how about quarterly pit-stops as well? Sounds as if you might need them.

Well-being all the way

Let's get back to the present, to your 60s. It's your great opportunity – the beginning of the rest of your life. Keeping active and staying active, getting fitter and taking care of your body, mind and mood, will improve your health and well-being. Being true to yourself, but open and connected with others, will help you thrive and build resilience. You need to nurture your relationships as well as take care of your bits, both are important. Try to spread your happiness when you find it, it will be infectious. Life needs 'being' and 'doing', focusing on the present, learning from the past, and planning for the future.

We hope that this advice will be useful and that following it, where appropriate for you, will enhance your well-being, help you prevent the preventable and manage conditions you may already have. And you have your own resources too, and a lifetime's experience to build on and to share, generously, with others.

Resilience and well-being help you cope with the stuff of life when it comes along. You are the navigator and you're steering the direction of your life. So Sod 60! Live your life to the full.

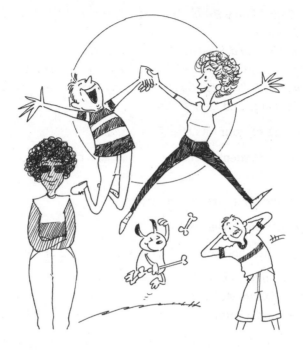

Further reading

Dear Readers, you may find the following books useful. We discussed good, reliable online information sources in Chapter 8 (see page 203). NHS Choices (www.nhs.uk) is a golden resource for every aspect of health care and well-being you could think of. It is regularly updated, and worth looking at whenever you have a problem or need advice or links to other sources of help.

Here are some books …

… on getting older:

- *Being Mortal: Illness, Medicine and What Matters in the End* by Atul Gawande.

- *The Virginia Monologues: Why Growing Old is Great* by Virginia Ironside.
- *You're Looking Very Well: The Surprising Nature of Getting Old* by Lewis Wolpert.

... for your mind and mood:

- *Rainy Brain, Sunny Brain: The New Science of Optimism and Pessimism* by Elaine Fox.
- *Thinking, Fast and Slow* by Daniel Kahneman.
- *The Aging Mind: An Owner's Manual* by Patrick Rabbit.
- *Mindfulness: A Practical Guide to Finding Peace in a Frantic World* by Mark Williams and Danny Penman.

...for taking care of your bits (and Rhythm and Blues):

- A Guide to Women's Health: Fifty and Forward, a report by Celeste Robb-Nicholson.

... for coping with Stuff, the mindful way:

- *Full Catastrophe Living* by Kabat-Zinn.

... for being a carer, and coping with dementia in the family:

- *When a Family Member Has Dementia (Steps to Becoming a Resilient Carer)* by Susan McCurry.
- *Keeping Mum, Caring for Someone with Dementia* by Marianne Talbot.

... on the benefits of physical activity, healthy lifestyle and Mediterranean diet:

- 'Physical activity predicts gray matter volume in late adulthood' by K.I. Erickson for The Cardiovascular Health Study. Published in the journal Neurology.
- 'An investigation into the relationship between age and physiological function in highly active older adults' by Pollock Ross. Published online in the Journal of Physiology.
- 'Healthy diet and lifestyle and risk of stroke in a prospective cohort of women' by S.C. Larsson. Published in the journal Neurology.
- 'Mediterranean dietary pattern and primary prevention of cardiovascular disease' by K. Rees. Published in the Cochrane Database Systematic Review.

ACKNOWLEDGEMENTS

Most of all, we would like to thank our patients, who have taught us what our textbooks didn't!

Many colleagues have been generous with their time and, in particular, we would like to thank the following clinicians and scientists for helpful discussions, advice, or comments on parts of the text: Julie Anderson, Caroline Champagne, Andy Chivers, Robert Clarke, Rory Collins, James Edwards, Sally Hope, Tess McPherson, Jeremy Noble, Morwyn Porter, Jane Roblin and Helen Steel. But we claim full responsibility for all the errors and omissions in the content of this book, and hope there aren't too many.

We would also like to thank Marion Foster, Ewart Cockram, Susie, Marianne Talbot, Ann Marie's sons and friends, and others who didn't want to be named, for advice or contributions from their personal experience.

On the publishing side, Charlotte Croft has provided invaluable suggestions, support and input at every step. And thanks to Sarah Connelly and colleagues for essential editorial skills and guidance.

David Mostyn has done wonderful drawings, putting into pictures what would take pages more to say.

Last but by no means least, we thank our families and friends for cheerfully putting up with us! Particular thanks to Tom Cockram, for interesting thoughts on the science of ageing, to Lucy Parker for constructive comments at so many stages, and to Ewart and Joy Cockram, for unfailing support and wisdom.

INDEX